Sweet Delicacies of the Mediterranean Sea

Mediterranean Desserts and Treats to
Satisfy Your Sweet Tooth

By
Delia Bell

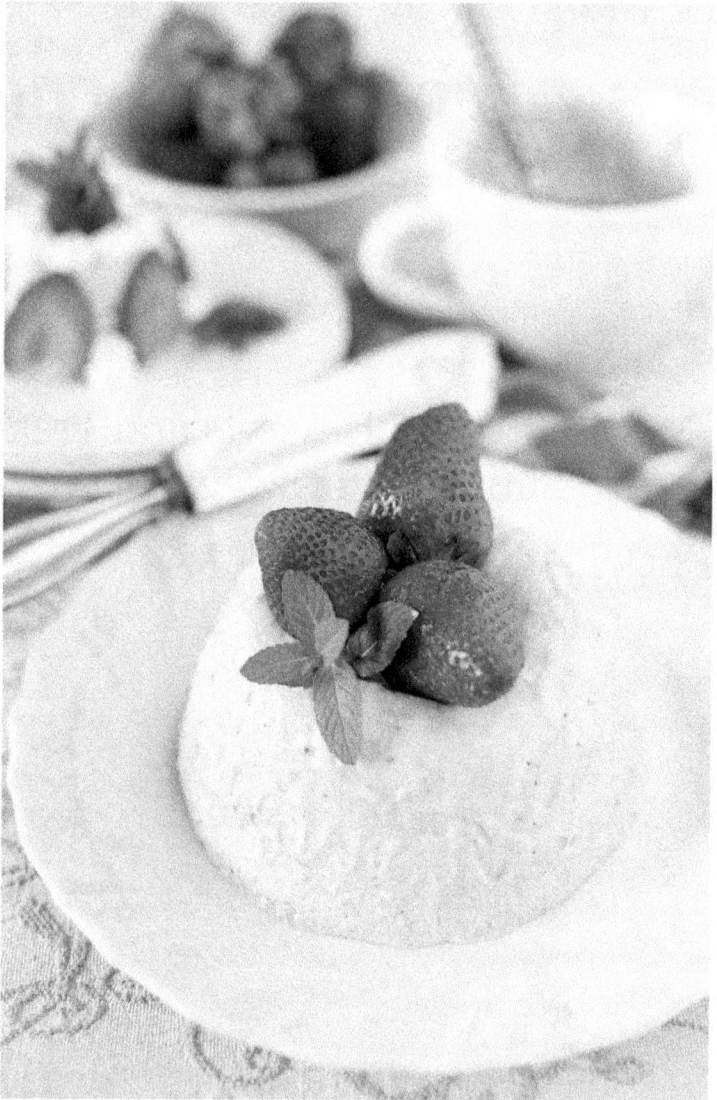

Table of Contents

INTRODUCTION

What is the Mediterranean Diet?

The Mediterranean diet is based on the diets of traditional eating habits from the 1960s of people from countries that surround the Mediterranean Sea, such as Greece, Italy, and Spain, and it encourages the consumption of fresh, seasonal, and local foods. The Mediterranean diet has become popular because individuals show low rates of heart disease, chronic disease, and obesity. The Mediterranean diet profile focuses on whole grains, good fats (fish, olive oil, nuts etc.), vegetables, fruits, fish, and very low consumption of any non-fish meat. Along with food, the Mediterranean diet emphasizes the need to spend time eating with family and physical activity. The Mediterranean diet is not a single prescribed diet, but rather a general food-based eating pattern, which is marked by local and cultural differences throughout the Mediterranean region.

The diet is generally characterized by a high intake of plant-based foods (e.g. fresh fruit and vegetables, nuts, and cereals) and olive oil, a moderate intake of fish and poultry, and low intakes of dairy products (mostly yoghurt and cheese), red and processed meats, and sweets. Wine is typically consumed in moderation and, normally, with a meal. A strong focus is placed on social and cultural aspects, such as communal mealtimes, resting after eating, and regular physical activity. Nowadays, however, the diet is no longer followed as widely as it was 30-50 years ago, as the diets of people living in these regions are becoming more 'Westernized' and higher in energy dense foods.

Benefits

The Mediterranean diet is not a weight loss, but increasing fiber intake and cutting out red meat, animal fats, and processed food may lead to weight loss. People who follow the diet may also have a lower risk of various diseases.

Heart health

In the 1950s, an American scientist, found that people living in the poorer areas of southern Italy had a lower risk of heart disease and death than those in wealthier parts of New York. Dr. Keys attributed this to diet. Since then, many studies have indicated that following a Mediterranean diet can help the body maintain healthy cholesterol levels and reduce the risk of high blood pressure and cardiovascular disease. The overall pattern of the Mediterranean diet is similar to their own dietary recommendations. A high proportion of calories on the diet come from fat, which can increase the risk of obesity. However, they also note that this fat is mainly unsaturated, which makes it a more healthful option than that from the typical American diet.

Protection from disease
The Mediterranean diet focuses on plant-based foods, and these are good sources of antioxidants.

The Mediterranean diet might offer protection from various cancers, and especially colorectal cancer. The reduction in risk may stem from the high intake of fruits, vegetables, and whole grains. By sticking to Mediterranean meals, people's levels of blood glucose and fats had decreased. During this time, there was also a lower incidence of stroke.

Diabetes
The Mediterranean diet may help prevent type 2 diabetes and improve markers of diabetes in people who already have the condition. Various other studies have concluded

that following the Mediterranean diet can reduce the risk of type 2 diabetes and cardiovascular disease, which often occur together.

Food to eat

There is no single definition of the Mediterranean diet, but one group of scientists used the following as their 2015 basis of research.

Vegetables: Include 3 to 9 servings a day.

Fresh fruit: Up to 2 servings a day.

Cereals: Mostly whole grain from 1 to 13 servings a day.

Oil: Up to 8 servings of extra virgin (cold pressed) olive oil a day.

Fat — mostly unsaturated — made up 37% of the total calories. Unsaturated fat comes from plant sources, such as olives and avocado. The Mediterranean diet also provided 33 grams (g) of fiber a day. The baseline diet for this study provided around 2,200 calories a day. Typical ingredients. Here are some examples of ingredients that people often include in the Mediterranean diet.

Vegetables: Tomatoes, peppers, onions, eggplant, zucchini, cucumber, leafy green vegetables, plus others.

Fruits: Melon, apples, apricots, peaches,

oranges, and lemons, and so on.

Legumes: Beans, lentils, and chickpeas.

Nuts and seeds: Almonds, walnuts, sunflower seeds, and cashews.

Unsaturated fat: Olive oil, sunflower oil, olives, and avocados.

Dairy products: Cheese and yogurt are the main dairy foods.

Cereals: These are mostly whole grain and include wheat and rice with bread accompanying many meals.

Fish: Sardines and other oily fish, as well as oysters and other shellfish. Poultry: Chicken or turkey.

Eggs: Chicken, quail, and duck eggs.

Drinks: A person can drink red wine in moderation.

The Mediterranean diet does not include strong liquor or carbonated and sweetened drinks. According to one definition, the diet limits red meat and sweets to less than 2 servings per week.

Food to avoid
Here's a list of foods you should generally limit while eating Mediterranean-style meals. Heavily processed

foods. Let's be real: Many, many foods are processed to some degree. A can of beans has been processed, in the sense that the beans have been cooked before being canned. Olive oil has been processed, because olives have been turned into oil. But when we talk about limiting processed foods, this really means avoiding things like frozen meals with tons of sodium. You should also limit soda, desserts and candy. As the adage goes, if the ingredient list includes items that your great-grandparents wouldn't recognize as food, it's probably processed. If you're buying a packaged food that's as close to its whole-food form as possible — such as frozen fruit or veggies with nothing added — you're good to go.

Processed red meat

On the Mediterranean diet, you should minimize your intake of red meat, such as steak. What about processed red meat, such as hot dogs and bacon? You should avoid these foods or limit them as much as possible. A study published in BMJ found that regularly eating red meat, especially processed varieties, was associated with a higher risk of death. Butter. Here's another food that should be limited on the Mediterranean diet. Use olive oil instead, which has many heart health benefits and contains less saturated fat than butter. According to the USDA National Nutrient Database, butter has 7 grams of saturated fat per tablespoon, while olive oil has about 2 grams.

Refined grains

The Mediterranean diet is centered around whole grains, such as farro, millet, couscous and brown rice. With this eating style, you'll generally want to limit your intake of refined grains such as white pasta and white bread.

Alcohol

When you're following the Mediterranean diet, red wine should be your chosen alcoholic drink. This is because red wine offers health benefits, particularly for the heart. But it's important to limit intake of any type of alcohol to up to one drink per day for women, as well as men older than 65, and up to two drinks daily for men age 65 and younger. The amount that counts as a drink is 5 ounces of wine, 12 ounces of beer or 1.5 ounces of 80-proof liquor.

Strawberry And Avocado Medley

Servings: 4

Cooking Time: 5 Minutes

Ingredients:

- 2 cups strawberry, halved
- 1 avocado, pitted and sliced
- 2 tablespoons slivered almonds

Directions:

1. Place all Ingredients: in a mixing bowl.

2. Toss to combine.

3. Allow to chill in the fridge before serving.

Nutrition Info: Calories per serving: 107; Carbs: 9.9g; Protein: 1.6g; Fat: 7.8g

Creamy Mint Strawberry Mix

Servings: 6

Cooking Time: 30 Minutes

Ingredients:

- Cooking spray
- ¼ cup stevia
- 1 and ½ cup almond flour
- 1 teaspoon baking powder
- 1 cup almond milk
- 1 egg, whisked
- 2 cups strawberries, sliced
- 1 tablespoon mint, chopped
- 1 teaspoon lime zest, grated
- ½ cup whipping cream

Directions:

1. In a bowl, combine the almond with the strawberries, mint and the other ingredients except the cooking spray and whisk well.

2. Grease 6 ramekins with the cooking spray, pour the strawberry mix inside, introduce in the oven and bake at 350 degrees F for 30 minutes.

3. Cool down and serve.

Nutrition Info: calories 200, fat 6.3, fiber 2, carbs 6.5, protein 8

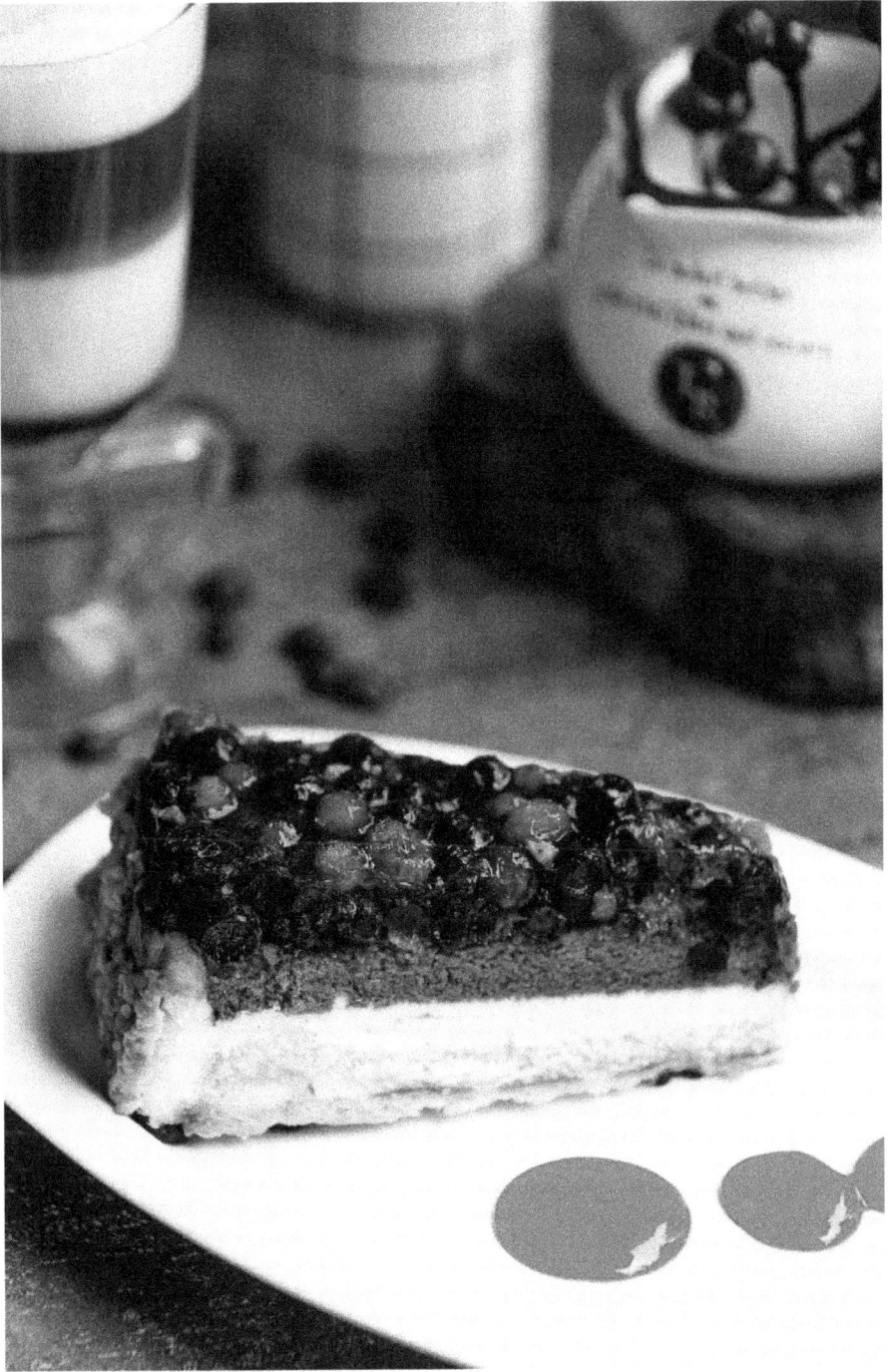

Creamy Pie

Servings: 6

Cooking Time: 30 Minutes

Ingredients:

- ¼ cup lemon juice
- 1 cup cream
- 4 egg yolks
- 4 tablespoons Erythritol
- 1 tablespoon cornstarch
- 1 teaspoon vanilla extract
- 3 tablespoons butter
- 6 oz wheat flour, whole grain

Directions:

1. Mix up together wheat flour and butter and knead the soft dough.

2. Put the dough in the round cake mold and flatten it in the shape of pie crust.

3. Bake it for 15 minutes at 365F.

4. Meanwhile, make the lemon filling: Mix up together cream, egg yolks, and lemon juice. When the liquid is smooth, start to heat it up over the medium heat. Stir it constantly.

5. When the liquid is hot, add vanilla extract, cornstarch, and Erythritol. Whisk well until smooth.

6. Bring the lemon filling to boil and remove it from the heat.

7. Cool it to the room temperature.

8. Cook the pie crust to the room temperature.

9. Pour the lemon filling over the pie crust, flatten it well and leave to cool in the fridge for 25 minutes.

Nutrition Info:Per Serving:calories 225, fat 11.4, fiber 0.8, carbs 34.8, protein 5.2

Watermelon Ice Cream

Servings: 2

Cooking Time: 5 Minutes

Ingredients:

- 8 oz watermelon
- 1 tablespoon gelatin powder

Directions:

1. Make the juice from the watermelon with the help of the fruit juicer.

2. Combine together 5 tablespoons of watermelon juice and 1 tablespoon of gelatin powder. Stir it and leave for 5 minutes.

3. Then preheat the watermelon juice until warm, add gelatin mixture and heat it up over the medium heat until gelatin is dissolved.

4. Then remove the liquid from the heat and pout it in the silicone molds.

5. Freeze the jelly for 30 minutes in the freezer or for 4 hours in the fridge.

Nutrition Info:Per Serving:calories 46, fat 0.2, fiber 0.4, carbs 8.5, protein 3.7

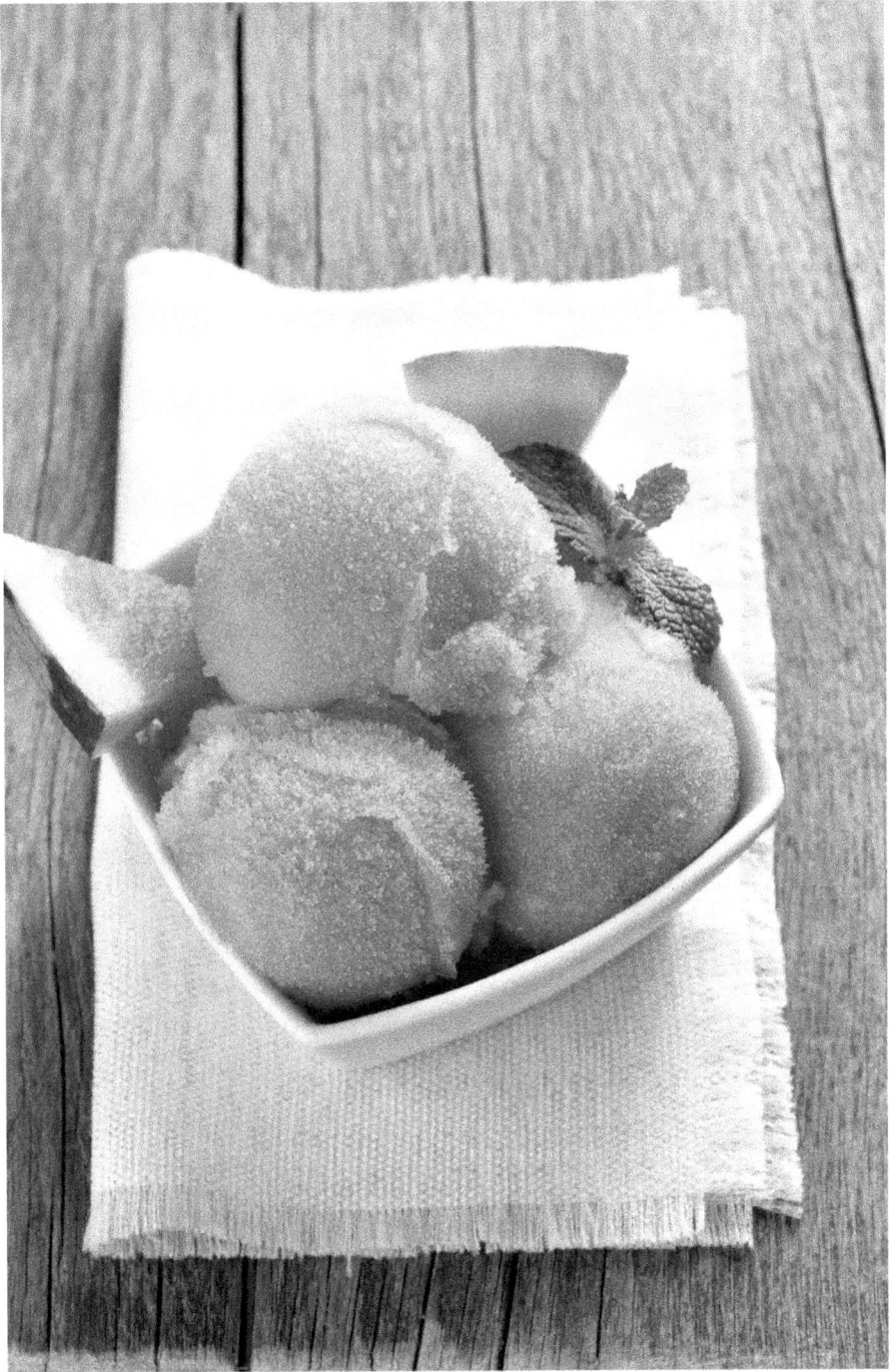

Hazelnut Pudding

Servings: 8

Cooking Time: 40 Minutes

Ingredients:

- 2 and ¼ cups almond flour
- 3 tablespoons hazelnuts, chopped
- 5 eggs, whisked
- 1 cup stevia
- 1 and 1/3 cups Greek yogurt
- 1 teaspoon baking powder
- 1 teaspoon vanilla extract

Directions:

1. In a bowl, combine the flour with the hazelnuts and the other ingredients, whisk well, and pour into a cake pan lined with parchment paper,
2. Introduce in the oven at 350 degrees F, bake for 30 minutes, cool down, slice and serve.

Nutrition Info: calories 178, fat 8.4, fiber 8.2, carbs 11.5, protein 1.4

Mediterranean Cheesecakes

Servings: 1 Cheesecake

Cooking Time: 20 Minutes

Ingredients:

- 4 cups shredded phyllo (kataifi dough)
- 1/2 cup butter, melted
- 12 oz. cream cheese
- 1 cup Greek yogurt
- 3/4 cup confectioners' sugar
- 1 TB. vanilla extract
- 2 TB. orange blossom water
- 1 TB. orange zest
- 2 large eggs
- 1 cup coconut flakes

Directions:

1. Preheat the oven to 450°F.

2. In a large bowl, and using your hands, combine shredded phyllo and melted butter, working the two together and breaking up phyllo shreds as you work.

3. Using a 12-cup muffin tin, add 1/3 cup shredded phyllo mixture to each tin, and press down to form crust

on the bottom of the cup. Bake crusts for 8 minutes, remove from the oven, and set aside.

4. In a large bowl, and using an electric mixer on low speed, blend cream cheese and Greek yogurt for 1 minute.

5. Add confectioners' sugar, vanilla extract, orange blossom water, and orange zest, and blend 1 minute.

6. Add eggs, and blend for about 30 seconds or just until eggs are incorporated.

7. Lightly coat the sides of each muffin tin with cooking spray.

8. Pour about 1/3 cup cream cheese mixture over crust in each tin. Do not overflow.

9. Bake for 12 minutes.

10. Spread shredded coconut on a baking sheet, and place in the oven with cheesecakes to toast for 4 or 5 minutes or until golden brown. Remove from the oven, and set aside.

11. Remove cheesecakes from the oven, and cool for 1 hour on the countertop.

12. Place the tin in the refrigerator, and cool for 1 more hour.

13. To serve, dip a sharp knife in warm water and then run it along the sides of cheesecakes to loosen from the

tin. Gently remove cheesecakes and place on a serving plate.

14. Sprinkle with toasted coconut flakes, and serve.

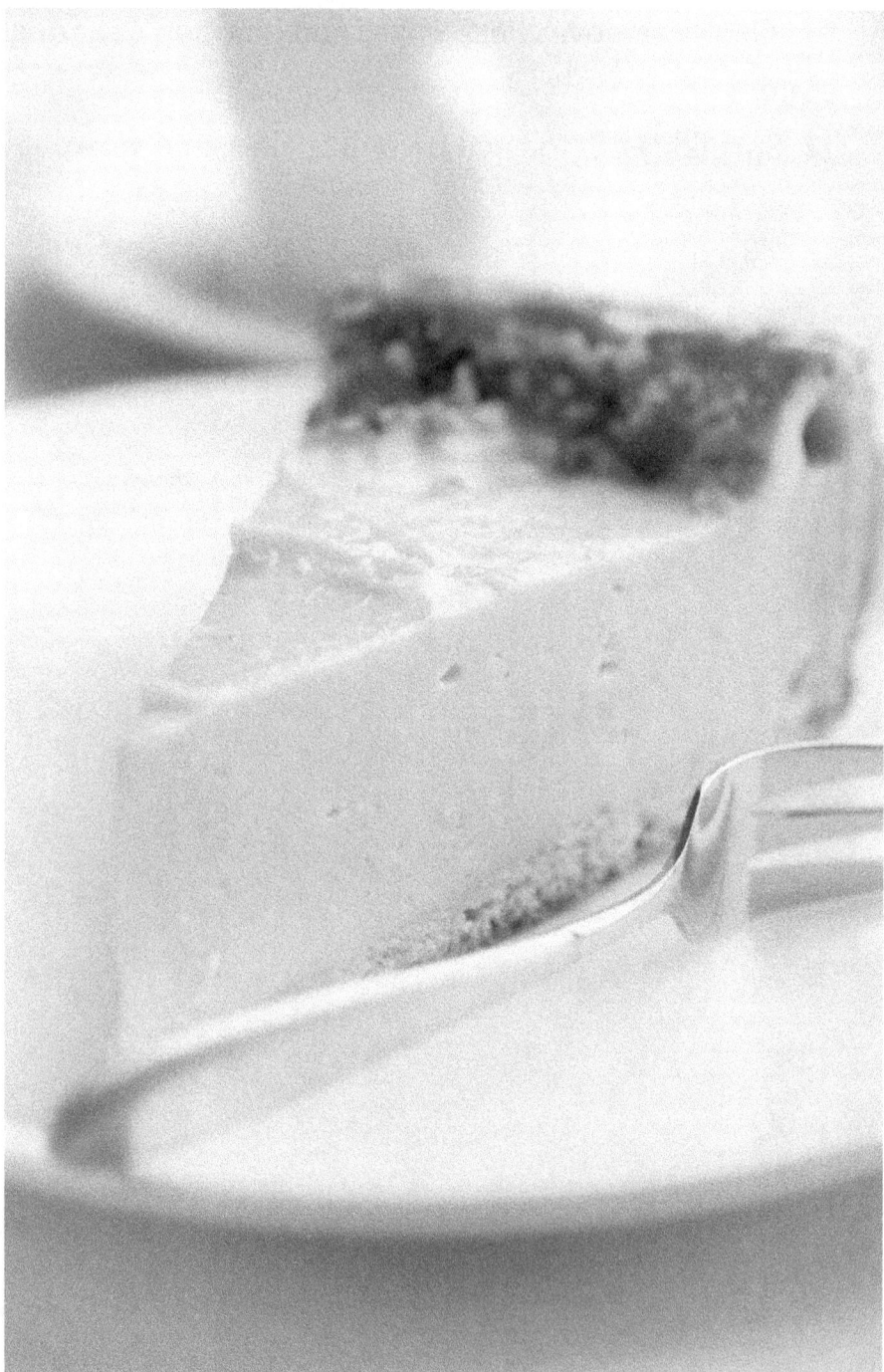

Melon Cucumber Smoothie

Servings: 2

Cooking Time: 5 Minutes

Ingredients:

- ½ cucumber
- 2 slices of melon
- 2 tablespoons lemon juice
- 1 pear, peeled and sliced
- 3 fresh mint leaves
- ½ cup almond milk

Directions:

1. Place all Ingredients: in a blender.

2. Blend until smooth.

3. Pour in a glass container and allow to chill in the fridge for at least 30 minutes.

Nutrition Info: Calories per serving: 253; Carbs: 59.3g; Protein: 5.7g; Fat: 2.1g

Mediterranean Style Fruit Medley

Servings: 7

Cooking Time: 5 Minutes

Ingredients:

- 4 fuyu persimmons, sliced into wedges
- 1 ½ cups grapes, halved
- 8 mint leaves, chopped
- 1 tablespoon lemon juice
- 1 tablespoon honey
- ½ cups almond, toasted and chopped

Directions:

1. Combine all Ingredients: in a bowl.
2. Toss then chill before serving.

Nutrition Info: Calories per serving:159; Carbs: 32g; Protein: 3g; Fat: 4g

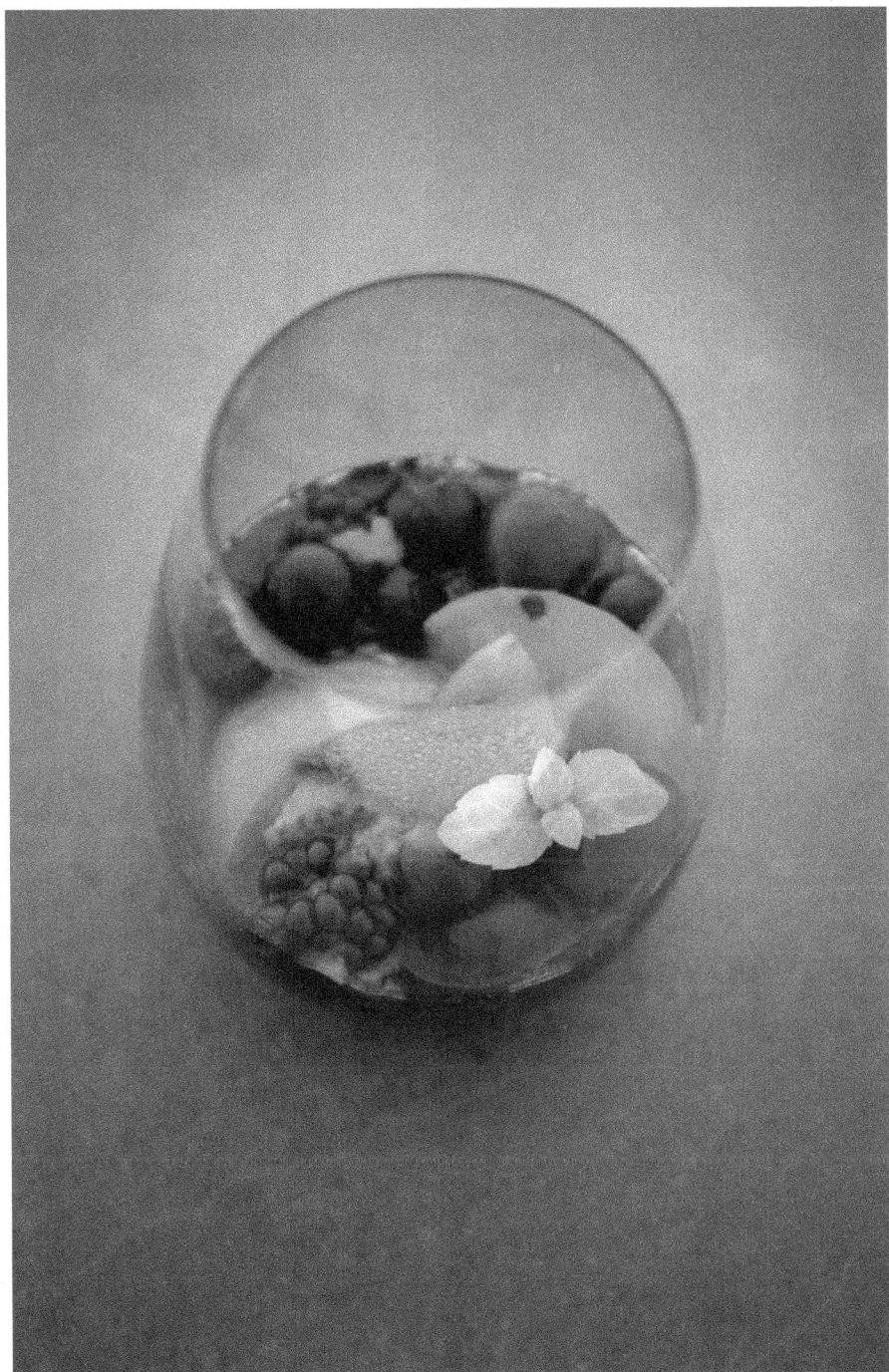

White Wine Grapefruit Poached Peaches

Servings: 6

Cooking Time: 40 Minutes

Ingredients:

- 4 peaches
- 2 cups white wine
- 1 grapefruit, peeled and juiced
- ¼ cup white sugar
- 1 cinnamon stick
- 1 star anise
- 1 cardamom pod
- 1 cup Greek yogurt for serving

Directions:

1. Combine the wine, grapefruit, sugar and spices in a saucepan.

2. Bring to a boil then place the peaches in the hot syrup.

3. Lower the heat and cover with a lid. Cook for 15 minutes then allow to cool down.

4. Carefully peel the peaches and place them in a small serving bowl.

5. Top with yogurt and serve right away.

Nutrition Info: Per Serving:Calories:157 Fat:0.9g
Protein:4.2g Carbohydrates:20.4g

Cinnamon Stuffed Peaches

Servings: 4

Cooking Time: 5 Minutes

Ingredients:
- 4 peaches, pitted, halved
- 2 tablespoons ricotta cheese
- 2 tablespoons of liquid honey
- ¾ cup of water
- ½ teaspoon vanilla extract
- ¾ teaspoon ground cinnamon
- 1 tablespoon almonds, sliced
- ¾ teaspoon saffron

Directions:

1. Pour water in the saucepan and bring to boil.

2. Add vanilla extract, saffron, ground cinnamon, and liquid honey.

3. Cook the liquid until the honey is melted.

4. Then remove it from the heat.

5. Put the halved peaches in the hot honey liquid.

6. Meanwhile, make the filling: mix up together ricotta cheese, vanilla extract, and sliced almonds.

7. Remove the peaches from honey liquid and arrange in the plate.

8. Fill 4 peach halves with ricotta filling and cover them with remaining peach halves.

9. Sprinkle the cooked dessert with liquid honey mixture gently.

Nutrition Info:Per Serving:calories 113, fat 1.8, fiber 2.8, carbs 23.9, protein 2.7

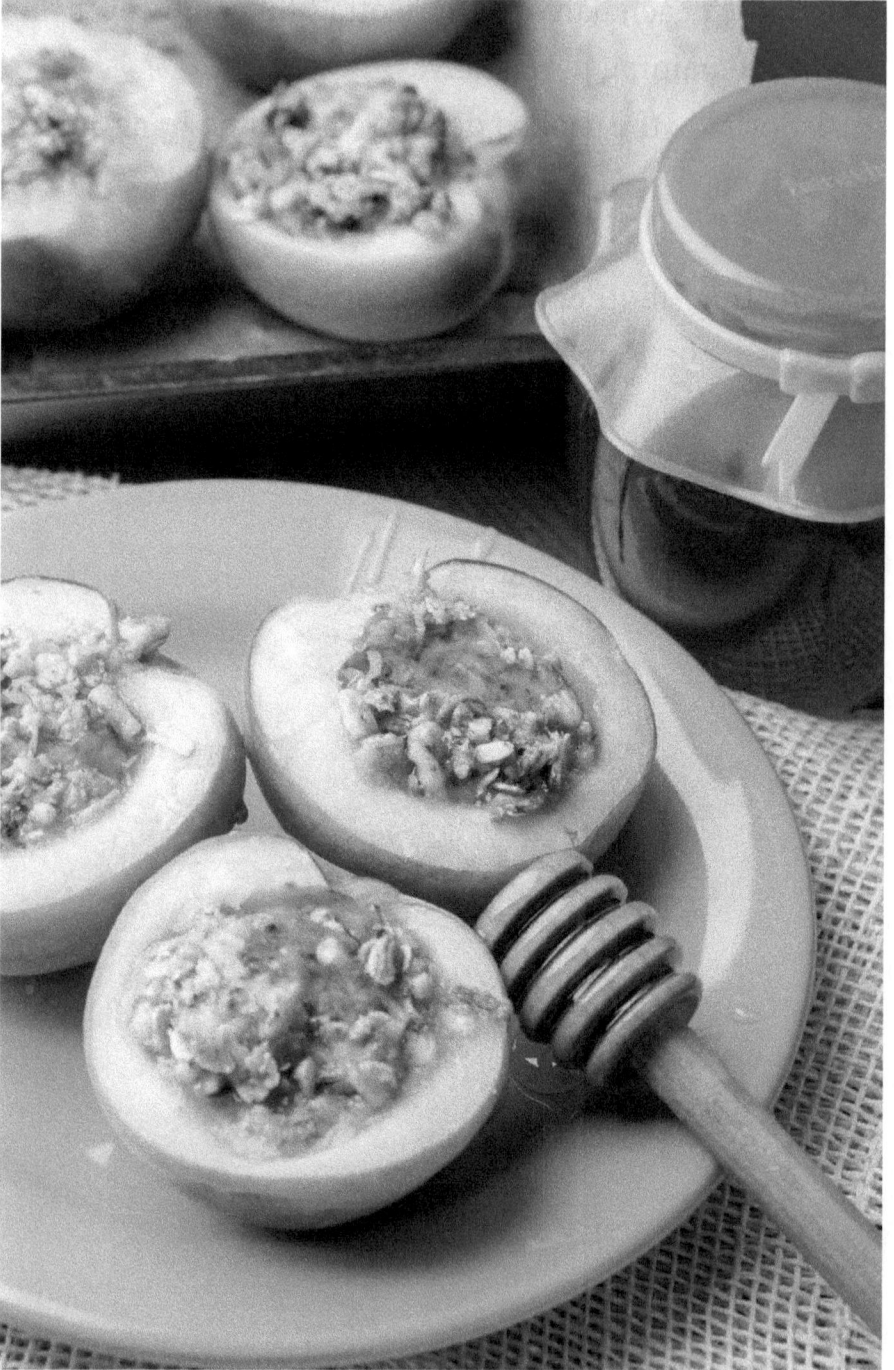

Eggless Farina Cake (namoura)

Servings: 1 Piece

Cooking Time: 40 Minutes

Ingredients:

- 2 cups farina
- 1/2 cup semolina
- 1/2 cup all-purpose flour
- 1 TB. baking powder
- 1 tsp. active dry yeast
- 1/2 cup sugar
- 1/2 cup plain Greek yogurt
- 1 cup whole milk
- 3/4 cup butter, melted
- 1/4 cup water
- 2 TB. tahini paste
- 15 almonds
- 2 cups Simple Syrup (recipe in Chapter 21)

Directions:

1. In a large bowl, combine farina, semolina, all-purpose flour, baking powder, yeast, sugar, Greek yogurt, whole milk, butter, and water. Set aside for 15 minutes.

2. Preheat the oven to 375°F.

3. Spread tahini paste evenly in the bottom of a 9×13-inch baking pan, and pour in cake batter. Arrange almonds on top of batter, about where each slice will be. Bake for 45 minutes or until golden brown.

4. Remove cake from the oven, and using a toothpick, poke holes throughout cake for Simple Syrup to seep into. Pour syrup over cake, and let cake sit for 1 hour to absorb syrup.

5. Cool cake completely before cutting and serving.

Mixed Berry Sorbet

Servings: 8

Cooking Time: 2 ½ Hours

Ingredients:

- 2 cups water
- ½ cup white sugar
- 2 cups mixed berries
- 1 tablespoon lemon juice
- 2 tablespoons honey
- 1 teaspoon lemon zest
- 1 mint sprig

Directions:

1. Combine the water, sugar, berries, lemon juice, honey and lemon zest in a saucepan.

2. Bring to a boil and cook on low heat for 5 minutes.

3. Add the mint sprig and remove off heat. Allow to infuse for 10 minutes then remove the mint.

4. Pour the syrup into a blender and puree until smooth and creamy.

5. Pour the smooth syrup into an airtight container and freeze for at least 2 hours.

6. Serve the sorbet chilled.

Nutrition Info: Per Serving:Calories:84 Fat:0.1g Protein:0.4g Carbohydrates:21.3g

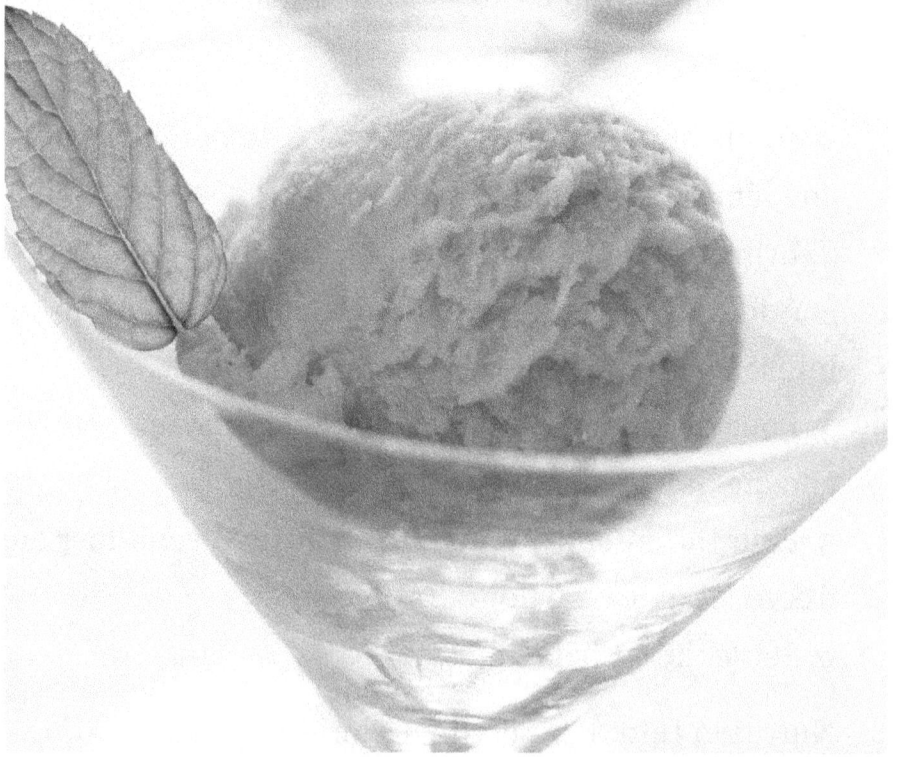

Almonds And Oats Pudding

Servings: 4

Cooking Time: 15 Minutes

Ingredients:

- 1 tablespoon lemon juice
- Zest of 1 lime
- 1 and ½ cups almond milk
- 1 teaspoon almond extract
- ½ cup oats
- 2 tablespoons stevia
- ½ cup silver almonds, chopped

Directions:

1. In a pan, combine the almond milk with the lime zest and the other ingredients, whisk, bring to a simmer and cook over medium heat for 15 minutes.
2. Divide the mix into bowls and serve cold.

Nutrition Info: calories 174, fat 12.1, fiber 3.2, carbs 3.9, protein 4.8

Banana And Berries Trifle

Servings: 10

Cooking Time: 5 Minutes

Ingredients:

- 8 oz biscuits, chopped
- ¼ cup strawberries, chopped
- 1 banana, chopped
- 1 peach, chopped
- ½ mango, chopped
- 1 cup grapes, chopped
- 1 tablespoon liquid honey
- 1 cup of orange juice
- ½ cup Plain yogurt
- ¼ cup cream cheese
- 1 teaspoon coconut flakes

Directions:

1. Bring the orange juice to boil and remove it from the heat.
2. Add liquid honey and stir until it is dissolved.
3. Cool the liquid to the room temperature.

4. Add chopped banana, peach, mango, grapes, and strawberries. Shake the fruits gently and leave to soak the orange juice for 15 minutes.

5. Meanwhile, with the help of the hand mixer mix up together Plain yogurt and cream cheese.

6. Then separate the chopped biscuits, yogurt mixture, and fruits in 4 parts.

7. Place the first part of biscuits in the big serving glass in one layer.

8. Spread it with yogurt mixture and add fruits.

9. Repeat the same steps till you use all ingredients.

10. Top the trifle with coconut flakes.

Nutrition Info:Per Serving:calories 164, fat 6.2, fiber 1.3, carbs 24.8, protein 3.2

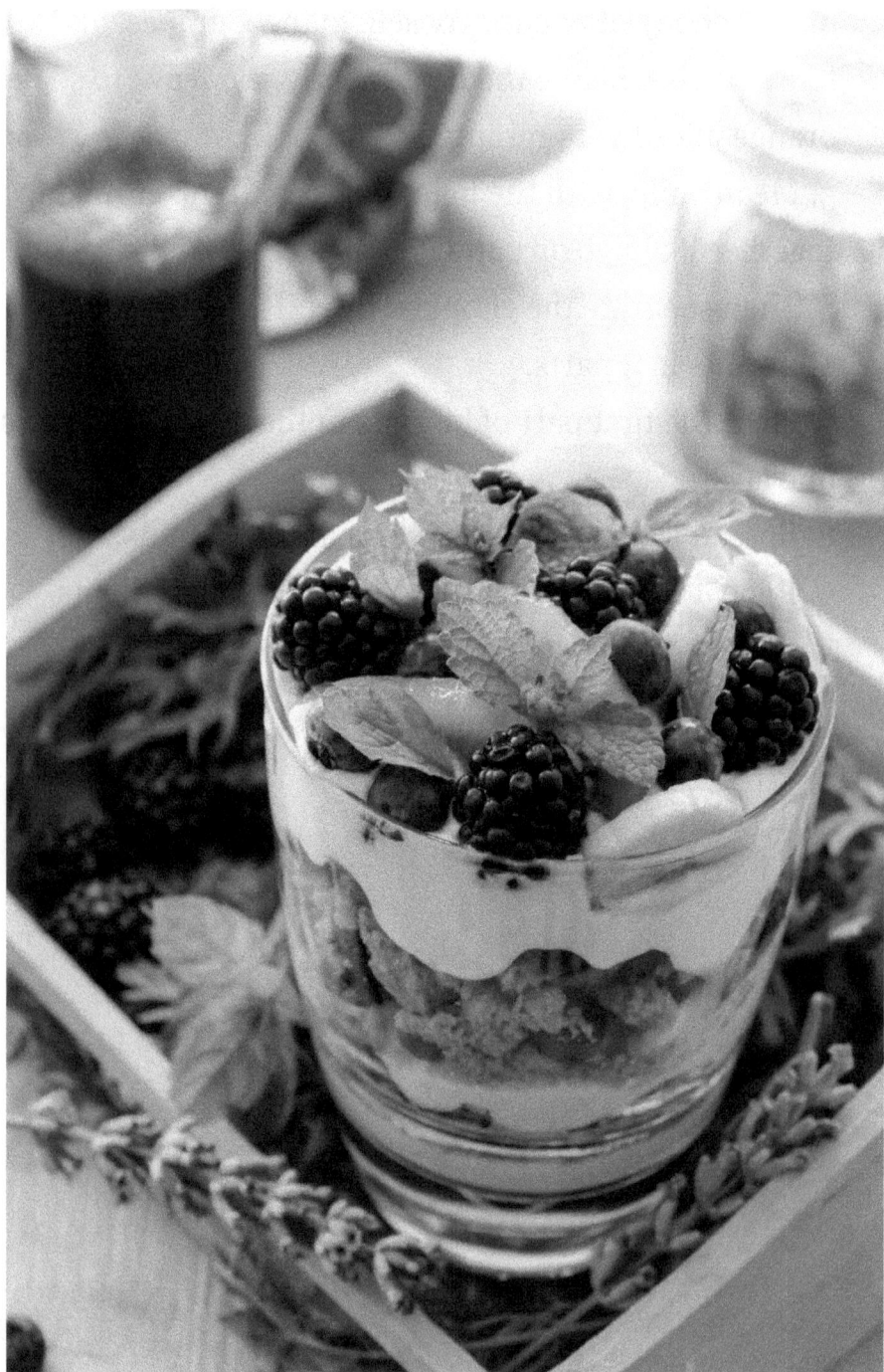

Chocolate Rice

Servings: 4

Cooking Time: 20 Minutes

Ingredients:

- 1 cup of rice
- 1 tbsp cocoa powder
- 2 tbsp maple syrup
- 2 cups almond milk

Directions:

1. Add all ingredients into the inner pot of instant pot and stir well.
2. Seal pot with lid and cook on high for 20 minutes.
3. Once done, allow to release pressure naturally for 10 minutes then release remaining using quick release. Remove lid.
4. Stir and serve.

Nutrition Info: Calories 474 Fat 29.1 g Carbohydrates 51.1 g Sugar 10 g Protein 6.3 g Cholesterol 0 mg

Lemon And Semolina Cookies

Servings: 6

Cooking Time: 20 Minutes

Ingredients:
- ½ teaspoon lemon zest, grated
- 4 tablespoons Erythritol
- 4 tablespoons semolina
- 2 tablespoons olive oil
- 8 tablespoons wheat flour, whole grain
- 1 teaspoon vanilla extract
- ½ teaspoon ground clove
- 3 tablespoons coconut oil
- ¼ teaspoon baking powder
- ¼ cup of water

Directions:

1. Make the dough: in the mixing bowl combine together lemon zest, semolina, olive oil, wheat flour, vanilla extract, ground clove, coconut oil, and baking powder.

2. Knead the soft dough.

3. Make the small cookies in the shape of walnuts and press them gently with the help of the fork.

4. Line the baking tray with the baking paper.

5. Place the cookies in the tray and bake them for 20 minutes at 375F.

6. Meanwhile, bring the water to boil.

7. Add Erythritol and simmer the liquid for 2 minutes over the medium heat. Cool it.

8. Pour the cooled sweet water over the hot baked cookies and leave them for 10 minutes.

9. When the cookies soak all liquid, transfer them in the serving plates.

Nutrition Info:Per Serving:calories 165, fat 11.7, fiber 0.6, carbs 23.7, protein 2

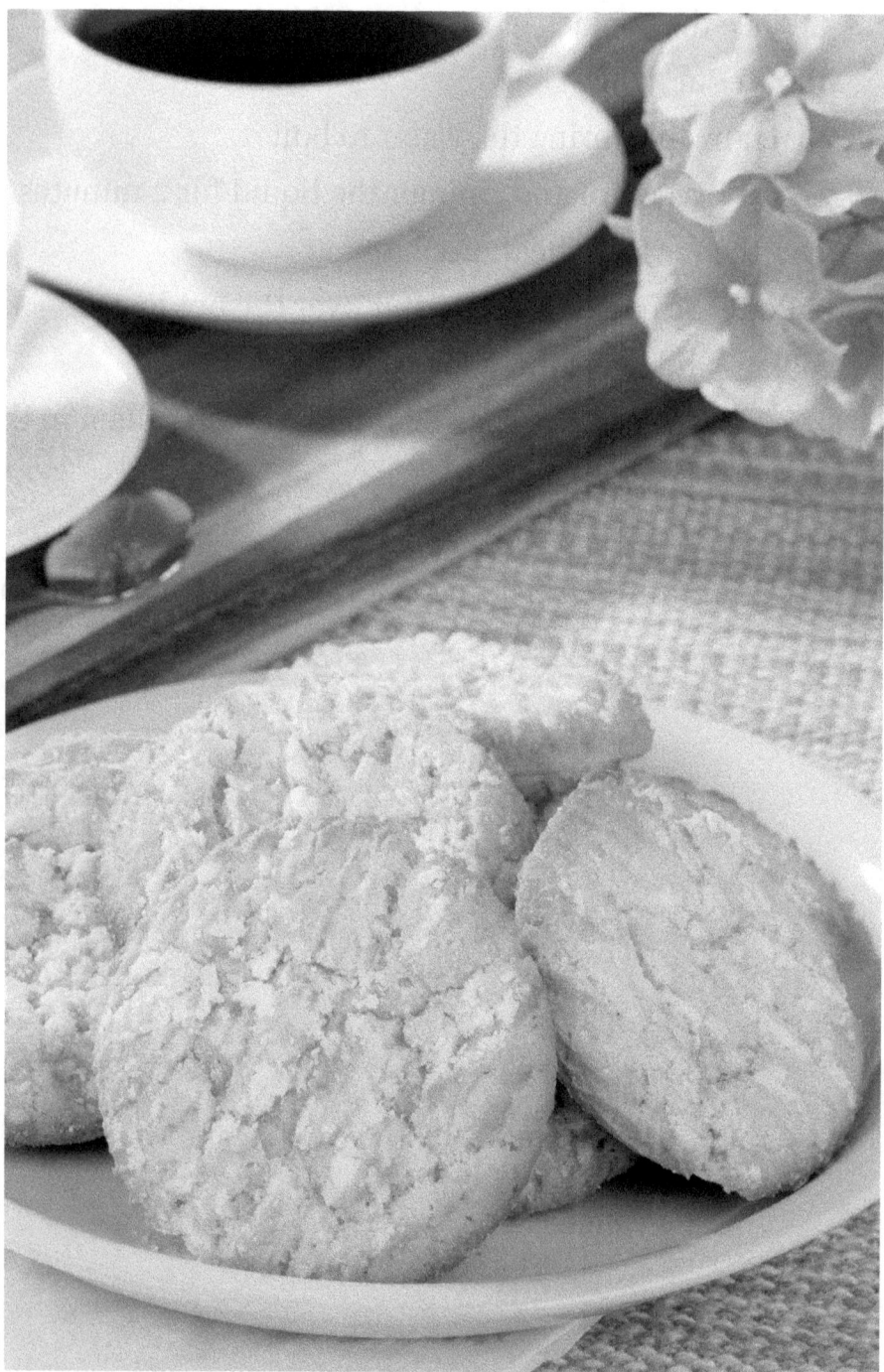

Strawberry Sorbet

Servings: 2

Cooking Time: 20 Minutes

Ingredients:

- 1 cup strawberries, chopped
- 1 tablespoon of liquid honey
- 2 tablespoons water
- 1 tablespoon lemon juice

Directions:

1. Preheat the water and liquid honey until you get homogenous liquid.

2. Blend the strawberries until smooth and combine them with honey liquid and lemon juice.

3. Transfer the strawberry mixture in the ice cream maker and churn it for 20 minutes or until the sorbet is thick.

4. Scoop the cooked sorbet in the ice cream cups.

Nutrition Info:Per Serving:calories 57, fat 0.3, fiber 1.5, carbs 14.3, protein 0.6

Halva (halawa)

Servings: ¼ Cup

Cooking Time: 10 Minutes

Ingredients:
- 11/2 cups honey
- 11/2 cups tahini paste
- 1 cup pistachios, coarsely chopped

Directions:

1. Pour honey into a saucepan, set over low heat, and bring to 240°F.

2. In another saucepan over low heat, bring tahini paste to 120°F.

3. In a bowl, whisk together heated honey and tahini paste until smooth. Fold in pistachios.

4. Line a loaf pan with parchment paper and spray with cooking spray. Pour tahini mixture into the loaf pan, and refrigerate for 2 days to set. 5. Cut halva into bite-size pieces, and serve.

Semolina Cake

Servings: 6

Cooking Time: 30 Minutes

Ingredients:

- ½ cup wheat flour, whole grain
- ½ cup semolina
- 1 teaspoon baking powder
- ½ cup Plain yogurt
- 1 teaspoon vanilla extract
- 4 tablespoons Erythritol
- 1 teaspoon lemon rind
- 2 tablespoons olive oil
- 1 tablespoon almond flakes
- 4 teaspoons liquid honey
- ½ cup of orange juice

Directions:

1. Mix up together wheat flour, semolina, baking powder, Plain yogurt, vanilla extract, Erythritol, and olive oil.

2. Then add lemon rind and mix up the ingredients until smooth.

3. Transfer the mixture in the non-sticky cake mold, sprinkle with almond flakes, and bake for 30 minutes at 365F.

4. Meanwhile, bring the orange juice to boil.

5. Add liquid honey and stir until dissolved.

6. When the cake is cooked, pour the hot orange juice mixture over it and let it rest for at least 10 minutes.

7. Cut the cake into the servings.

Nutrition Info:Per Serving:calories 179, fat 6.1, fiber 1.1, carbs 36.3, protein 4.5

Shredded Phyllo And Sweet Cheese Pie (knafeh)

Servings: 1/8 Pie

Cooking Time: 30 Minutes

Ingredients:

- 1 lb. pkg. shredded phyllo (kataifi dough)
- 1 cup butter, melted
- 1/2 cup whole milk
- 2 TB. semolina flour
- 1 lb. ricotta cheese
- 2 cups mozzarella cheese, shredded
- 2 TB. sugar
- 1 cup Simple Syrup (recipe later in this chapter)

Directions:

1. 1 cup Simple Syrup (recipe later in this chapter)
2. In a food processor fitted with a chopping blade, pulse shredded phyllo
and butter 10 times. Transfer mixture to a bowl.
3. In a small saucepan over low heat, warm whole milk.
4. Stir in semolina flour, and cook for 1 minute.

5. Rinse the food processor, and to it, add ricotta cheese, mozzarella cheese, sugar, and semolina mixture. Blend for 1 minute.

6. Preheat the oven to 375ºF.

7. In a 9-inch-round baking dish, add 1/2 of shredded phyllo mixture, and press down to compress. Add cheese mixture, and spread out evenly. Add rest of shredded phyllo mixture, spread evenly, and gently press down. Bake for 40 minutes or until golden brown.

8. Let pie rest for 10 minutes before serving with Simple Syrup drizzled over top.

Lemon Pear Compote

Servings: 6

Cooking Time: 15 Minutes

Ingredients:

- 3 cups pears, cored and cut into chunks
- 1 tsp vanilla
- 1 tsp liquid stevia
- 1 tbsp lemon zest, grated
- 2 tbsp lemon juice

Directions:

1. Add all ingredients into the inner pot of instant pot and stir well.

2. Seal pot with lid and cook on high for 15 minutes.

3. Once done, allow to release pressure naturally for 10 minutes then release remaining using quick release. Remove lid.

4. Stir and serve.

Nutrition Info: Calories 50 Fat 0.2 g Carbohydrates 12.7 g Sugar 8.1 g Protein 0.4 g Cholesterol 0 mg

Cinnamon Pear Jam

Servings: 12

Cooking Time: 4 Minutes

Ingredients:

- 8 pears, cored and cut into quarters
- 1 tsp cinnamon
- 1/4 cup apple juice
- 2 apples, peeled, cored and diced

Directions:

1. Add all ingredients into the inner pot of instant pot and stir well.
2. Seal pot with lid and cook on high for 4 minutes.
3. Once done, allow to release pressure naturally. Remove lid.
4. Blend pear apple mixture using an immersion blender until smooth.
5. Serve and enjoy.

Nutrition Info: Calories 103 Fat 0.3 g Carbohydrates 27.1 g Sugar 18 g Protein 0.6 g Cholesterol 0 mg

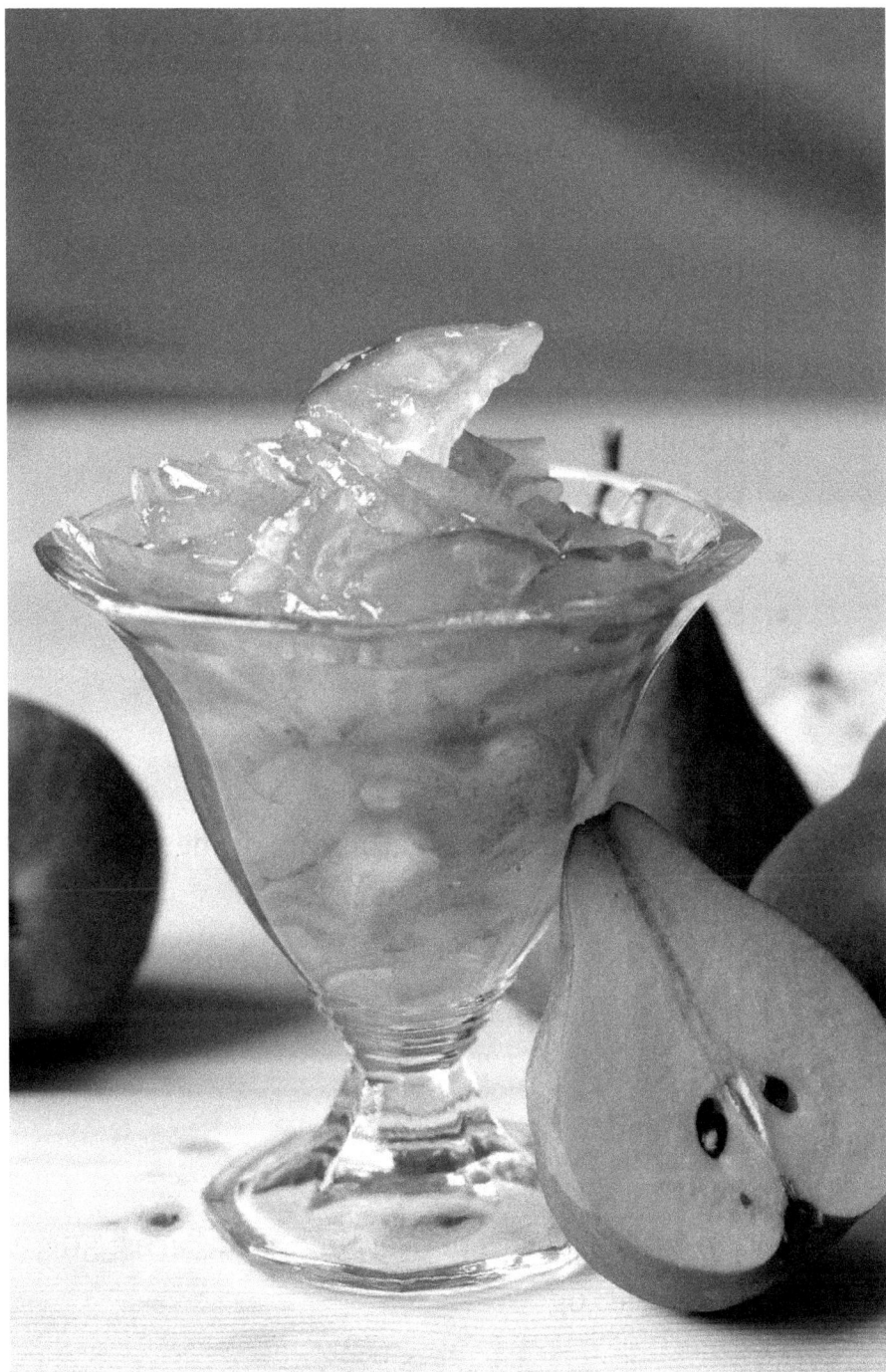

Apple And Walnut Salad

Servings: 6

Cooking Time: 5 Minutes

Ingredients:

- Juice from ½ orange
- Zest from ½ orange, grated
- 2 tablespoons honey
- 1 tablespoon olive oil
- 4 medium Gala apples, cubed
- 8 dried apricots, chopped
- ¼ cup walnuts, toasted and chopped

Directions:

1. In a small bowl, whisk together the orange juice, zest, honey, and olive oil. Set aside.
2. In a larger bowl, toss the apples, apricots, and walnuts.
3. Drizzle with the vinaigrette and toss to coat all Ingredients.
4. Serve chilled.

Nutrition Info: Calories per serving: 178; Carbs: 30g; Protein: 1g; Fat: 6g

Banana Kale Smoothie

Servings: 3

Cooking Time: 5 Minutes

Ingredients:

- 2 cups kale leaves
- 1 cup almond milk
- ½ cup crushed ice
- 1 banana, peeled
- 1 apple, peeled and cored
- A dash of cinnamon

Directions:

1. Place all Ingredients: in a blender.

2. Blend until smooth.

3. Pour in a glass container and allow to chill in the fridge for at least 30 minutes.

Nutrition Info: Calories per serving: 165; Carbs: 32.1g; Protein: 2.3g; Fat: 4.2g

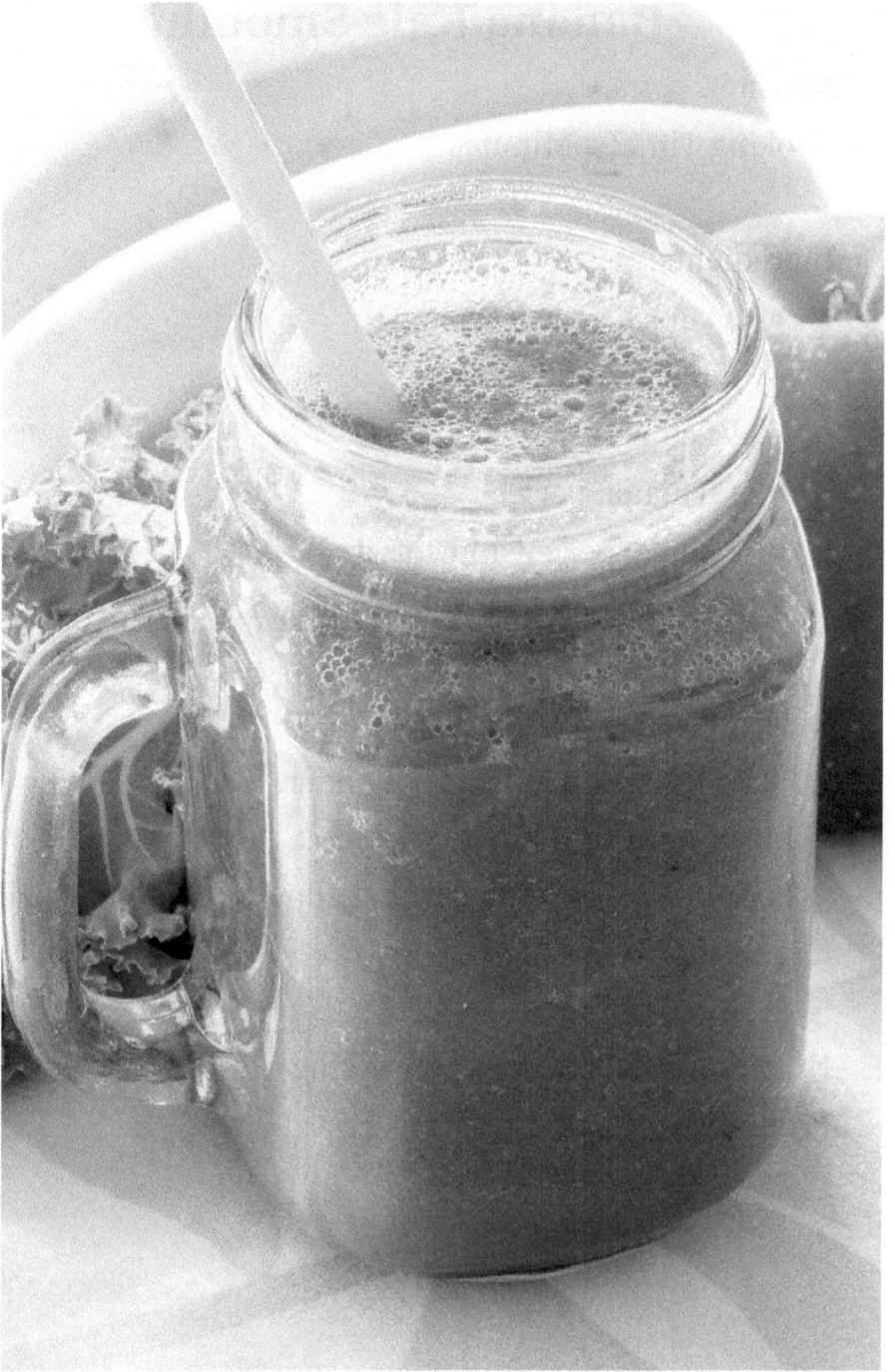

Phyllo Custard Pockets (shaabiyat)

Servings: 1 Pocket

Cooking Time: 10 Minutes

Ingredients:

- 8 phyllo sheets
- 1/2 cup butter, melted
- 21/4 cups Ashta Custard (recipe later in this chapter)
- 1 cup Simple Syrup (recipe later in this chapter)
- 1/2 cup pistachios, ground

Directions:

1. Preheat the oven to 450°F.

2. Lay out a sheet of phyllo dough, brush with butter, and layer another sheet of phyllo dough on top. Cut sheets into 3 equal-size columns, each about 3 or 4 inches wide.

3. Place 3 tablespoons Ashta Custard at one end of each column, and fold the bottom-right corner up and over custard. Pull up bottom-left corner, and repeat folding each corner up to the opposite corner, forming a triangle as you fold.

4. Place triangle pockets on a baking sheet, brush with butter, and bake for 10 minutes or until golden brown.

5. Serve warm or cold, drizzled with Simple Syrup and sprinkled with pistachios.

Chocolate Baklava

Servings: 4

Cooking Time: 35 Minutes

Ingredients:

- 24 sheets (14 x 9-inch) frozen whole-wheat phyllo (filo) dough, thawed 1/8 teaspoon salt
- 1/3 cup toasted walnuts, chopped coarsely
- 1/3 cup almonds, blanched toasted, chopped coarsely
- 1/2 teaspoon ground cinnamon
- 1/2 cup water
- 1/2 cup hazelnuts, toasted, chopped coarsely
- 1/2 cup pistachios, roasted, chopped coarsely
- 3/4 cup honey
- 1/2 cup of butter, melted
- 1 cup chocolate-hazelnut spread (I used Nutella)
- 1 piece (3-inch) cinnamon stick
- Cooking spray

Directions:
1. Into medium-sized saucepan, combine the water, honey, and the cinnamon stick; stir until the honey is dissolved. Increase the heat/flame to medium; continue

cooking for about 10 minutes without stirring. A candy thermometer should read 230F. Remove the saucepan from the heat and then keep warm. Remove and discard the cinnamon stick.

2. Preheat the oven to 350F.

3. Put the chocolate-hazelnut spread into microwavable bowl; microwave the spread for about 30 seconds on HIGH or until the spread is melted.

4. In a bowl, combine the hazelnuts, pistachios, almonds, walnuts, ground cinnamon, and the salt.

5. Lightly grease with the cooking spray a 9x13-inch ceramic or glass baking dish.

6. Put 1 sheet lengthwise into the bottom of the prepared baking dish, extending the ends of the sheet over the edges of the dish. Lightly brush the sheet with the butter. Repeat the process with 5 sheets phyllo and a light brush of butter. Drizzle 1/3 cup of the melted chocolate-hazelnut spread over the buttered phyllo sheets. Sprinkle about 1/3 of the nut mixture (1/2 cup) over the spread. Repeat the process, layering phyllo sheet, brush of butter, spread, and with nut mixture. For the last, nut mixture top layer, top with 6 phyllo sheets, pressing each phyllo gently into the dish and brushing each sheet with butter.

7. Slice the layers into 24 portions by making 3 cuts lengthwise and then 5 cuts crosswise with a sharp knife; bake for about 35 minutes at 350F or until the phyllo sheets are golden. Remove the dish from the oven, drizzle the honey sauce over the baklava. Pace the dish on a wire rack and let cool. Cover and store the baklavas at normal room temperature if not serving right away.

Nutrition Info:Per Serving:238 Cal, 13.4 g total fat (4.3 g sat. fat, 5.6 g mono fat, 2 g poly fat), 4 g protein, 27.8 g total carbs., 1.6 g fiber, 10 mg chol., 1.3 mg iron, 148 mg sodium, and 29 mg calcium.

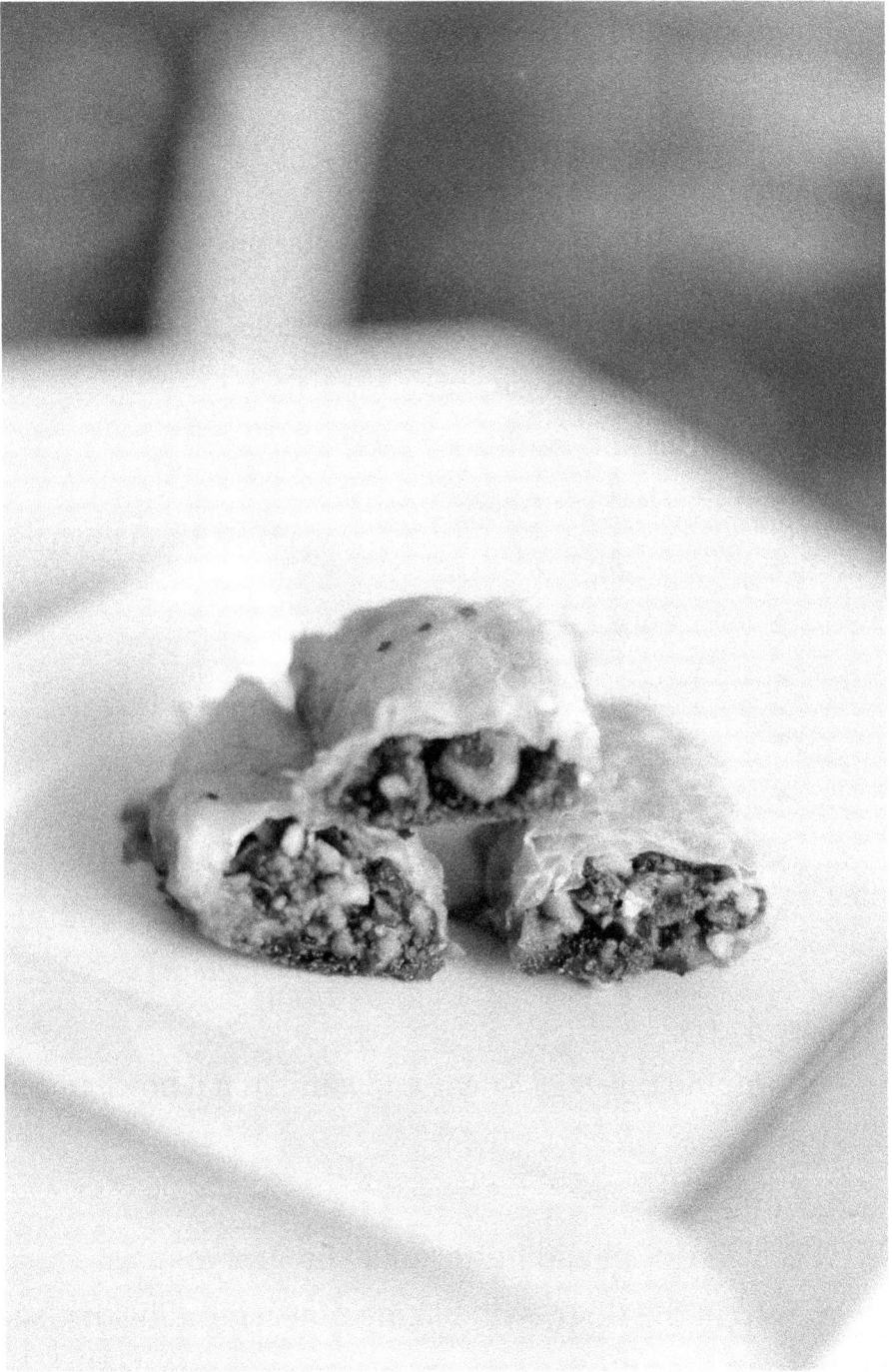

Apricot Rosemary Muffins

Servings: 12

Cooking Time: 1 Hour

Ingredients:

- 2 eggs
- 1/3 cup white sugar
- 1 teaspoon vanilla extract
- 1 cup buttermilk
- ¼ cup olive oil
- 1 ½ cups all-purpose flour
- ¼ teaspoon salt
- 1 teaspoon baking powder
- ¼ teaspoon baking soda
- 4 apricots, pitted and diced
- 1 teaspoon dried rosemary

Directions:

1. Combine the eggs, sugar and vanilla in a bowl and mix until double in
volume.
2. Stir in the oil and buttermilk and mix well.
3. Fold in the flour, salt, baking powder and baking soda then add the apricots and rosemary and mix gently.

4. Spoon the batter in a muffin tin lined with muffin papers and bake in the preheated oven at 350F for 20-25 minutes or until the muffins pass the toothpick test.

5. Serve the muffins chilled.

Nutrition Info: Per Serving:Calories:140 Fat:5.4g Protein:3.4g Carbohydrates:20.1g

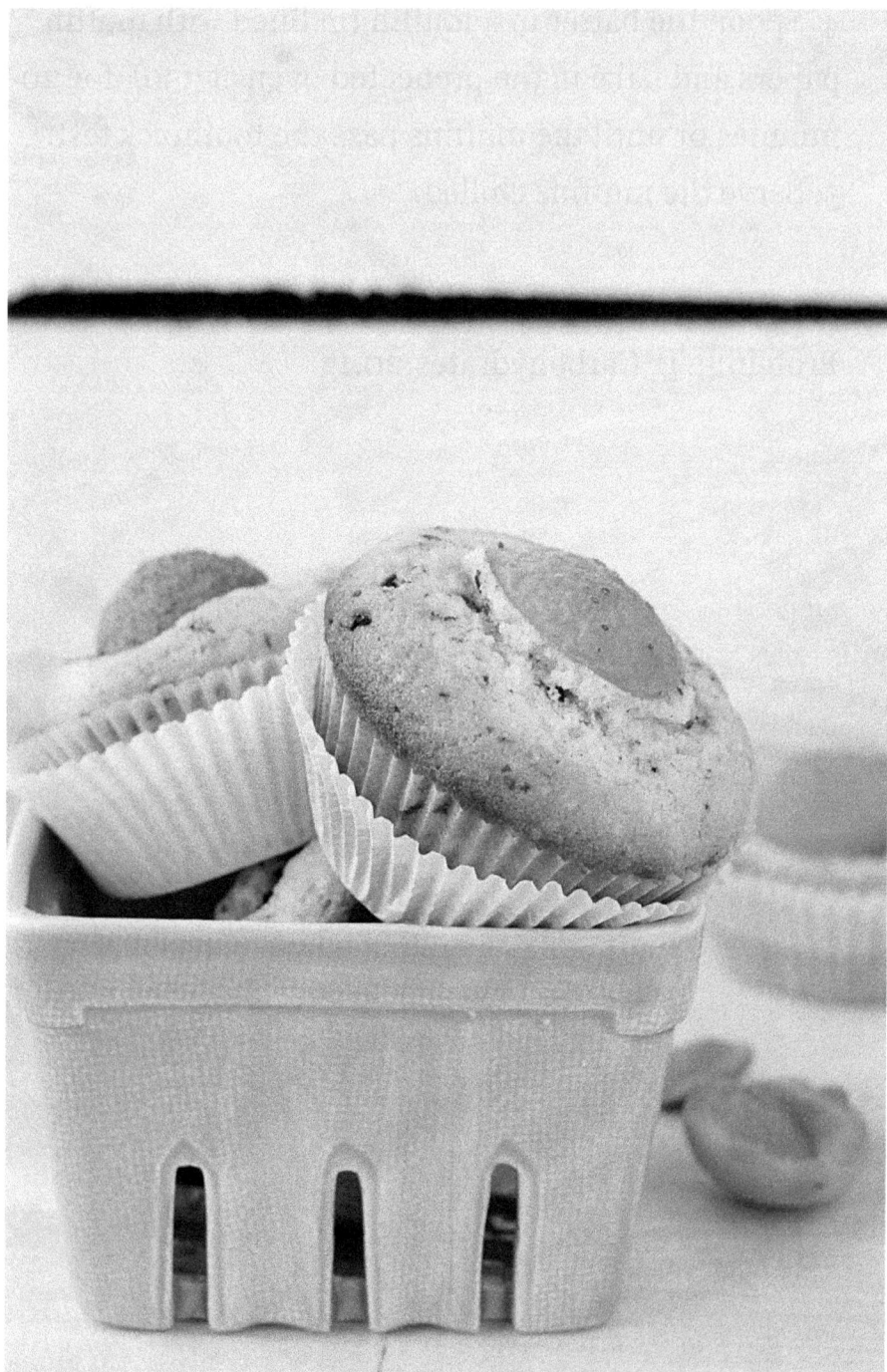

Blueberry Yogurt Mousse

Servings: 4

Cooking Time: 0 Minutes

Ingredients:

- 2 cups Greek yogurt
- ¼ cup stevia
- ¾ cup heavy cream
- 2 cups blueberries

Directions:

1. In a blender, combine the yogurt with the other ingredients, pulse well, divide into cups and keep in the fridge for 30 minutes before serving.

Nutrition Info: calories 141, fat 4.7, fiber 4.7, carbs 8.3, protein 0.8

Pistachio Cheesecake

Servings: 6

Cooking Time: 10 Minutes

Ingredients:

- ½ cup pistachio, chopped
- 4 teaspoons butter, softened
- 4 teaspoon Erythritol
- 2 cups cream cheese
- ½ cup cream, whipped

Directions:

1. Mix up together pistachios, butter, and Erythritol.

2. Put the mixture in the baking mold and bake for 10 minutes at 355F.

3. Meanwhile, whisk together cream cheese and whipped cream.

4. When the pistachio mixture is baked, chill it well.

5. After this, transfer the pistachio mixture in the round cake mold and flatten in one layer.

6. Then put the cream cheese mixture over the pistachio mixture, flatten the surface until smooth.

7. Cool the cheesecake in the fridge for 1 hour before serving.

Nutrition Info:Per Serving:calories 332, fat 33, fiber 0.5, carbs 7.4, protein 7

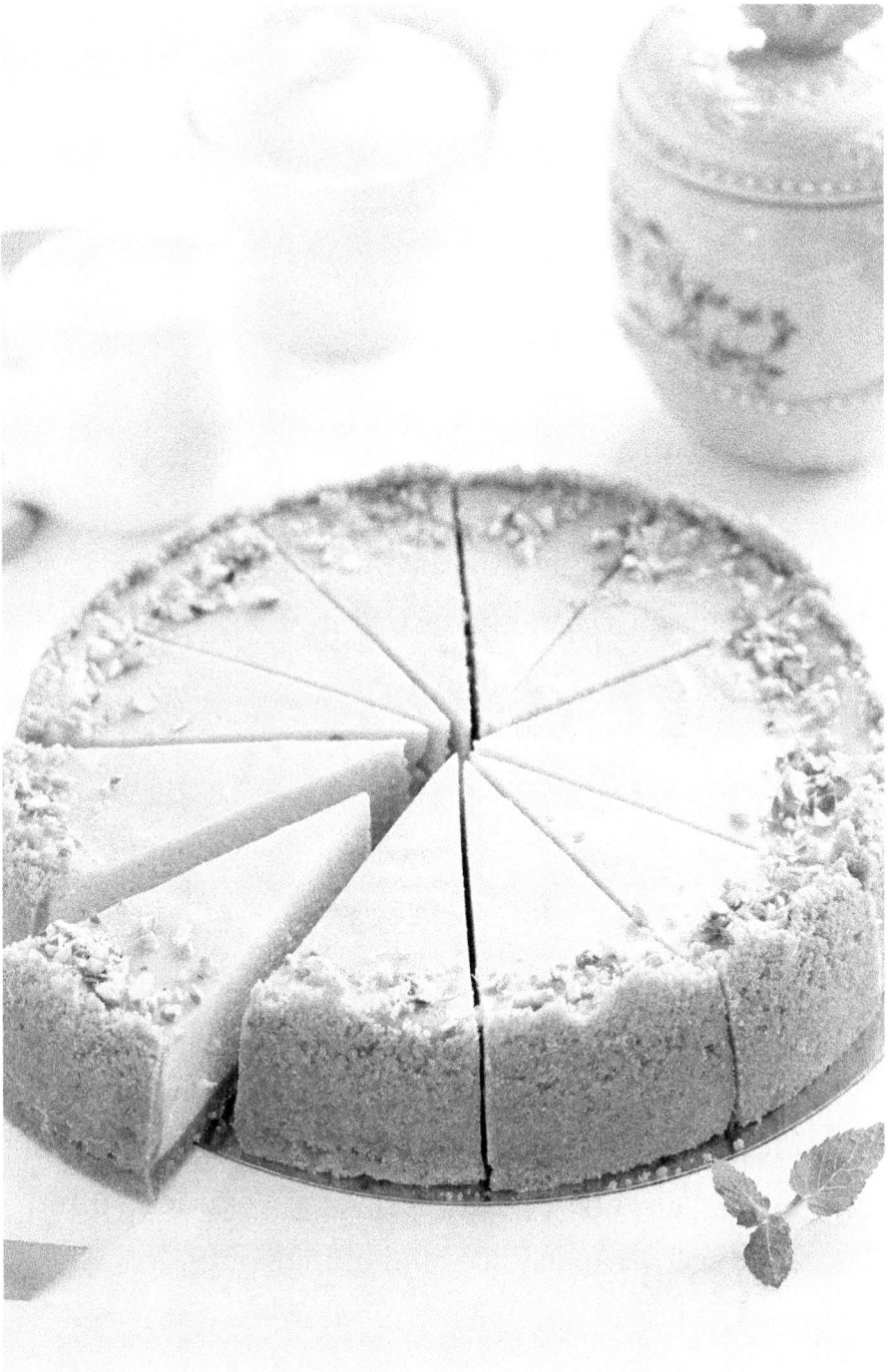

Almond Citrus Muffins

Servings: 6

Cooking Time: 30 Minutes

Ingredients:

- 2 eggs, beaten
- 1 ½ cup whole wheat flour
- ½ cup almond meal
- 1 teaspoon vanilla extract
- 1 tablespoon butter, softened
- 1 teaspoon orange zest, grated
- 1 tablespoon orange juice
- ¾ cup Erythritol
- 1 oz orange pulp
- 1 teaspoon baking powder
- ½ teaspoon lime zest, grated
- Cooking spray

Directions:

1. Make the muffin batter: combine together almond meal, eggs, whole wheat flour, vanilla extract, butter, orange zest, orange juice, and orange pulp.

2. Add lime zest and baking powder.

3. Then add Erythritol.

4. With the help of the hand mixer mix up the ingredients.

5. When the mixture is soft and smooth, it is done.

6. Spray the muffin molds with cooking spray from inside and preheat the oven to 365F.

7. Fill ½ part of every muffin mold with muffin batter and transfer them in the oven.

8. Cook the muffins for 30 minutes.

9. Then check if the muffins are cooked by piercing them with a toothpick (if it is dry, the muffins are cooked; if it is not dry, bake the muffins for 5-7 minutes more.)

Nutrition Info:Per Serving:calories 204, fat 7.7, fiber 1.9, carbs 57.1, protein 6.8

Mediterranean Bread Pudding (aish El Saraya)ad

Servings: 1/9 Of Pudding

Cooking Time: 20 Minutes

Ingredients:

- 8 slices white bread, crust removed
- 1 cup sugar
- 1/2 cup water
- 1 TB. fresh lemon juice
- 2 cups Simple Syrup (recipe later in this chapter)
- 4 cups Ashta Custard (recipe later in this chapter)
- 1/2 cup coconut flakes, toasted
- 1/2 cup pistachios, ground
- 1 strawberry, sliced

Directions:

1. Preheat the oven to 450°F.

2. Place slices of bread on a baking sheet, and toast for 10 minutes or until bread is golden brown and dry.

3. In a small saucepan over medium-low heat, combine sugar, water, and lemon juice. Simmer for 5 to 7 minutes or until sugar reaches a dark golden brown color.

4. Carefully pour hot dark brown syrup into an 8×8-inch baking dish, shifting the dish from side to side to spread syrup around bottom of dish.

5. Place 4 slices of bread on top of brown syrup. Pour 1 cup of Simple Syrup over bread, spread 2 cups Ashta Custard over bread, and add another layer of 4 slices of bread. Pour remaining 1 cup Simple Syrup over bread, and spread remaining 2 cups Ashta Custard over top bread layer.

6. Cover the dish with plastic wrap, and refrigerate for 4 hours.

7. Decorate top of dish with toasted coconut, pistachios, and strawberry slices, and serve.

Cinnamon Apple Rice Pudding

Servings: 8

Cooking Time: 15 Minutes

Ingredients:

- 1 cup of rice
- 1 tsp vanilla
- 1/4 apple, peeled and chopped
- 1/2 cup water
- 1 1/2 cup almond milk
- 1 tsp cinnamon
- 1 cinnamon stick

Directions:

1. Add all ingredients into the instant pot and stir well.

2. Seal pot with lid and cook on high for 15 minutes.

3. Once done, release pressure using quick release. Remove lid.

4. Stir and serve.

Nutrition Info: Calories 206 Fat 11.5 g Carbohydrates 23.7 g Sugar 2.7 g Protein 3 g Cholesterol 0 mg

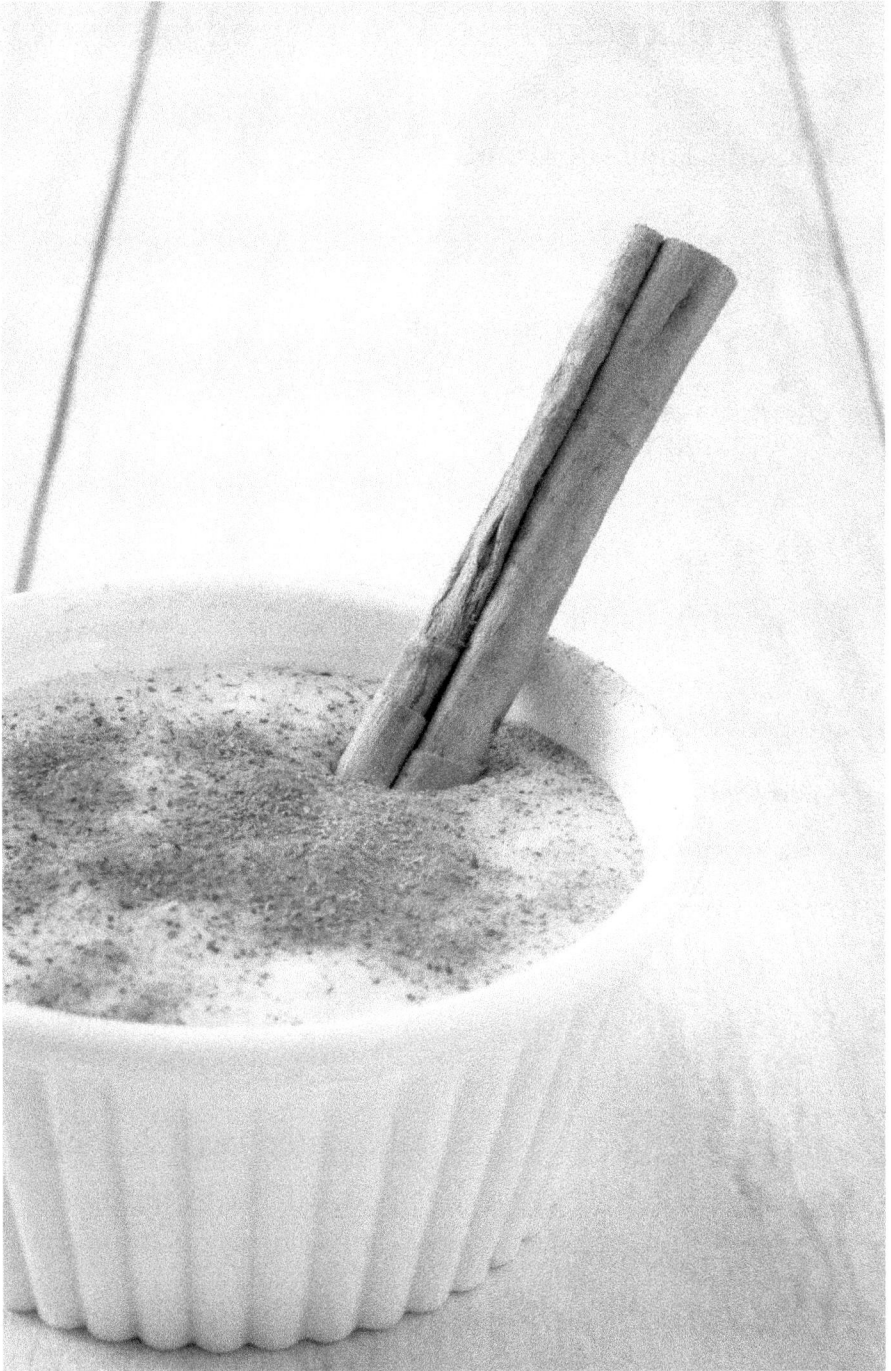

Custard-filled Pancakes (atayef)

Servings: 1 Pancake

Cooking Time: 15 Minutes

Ingredients:

- 1 cup all-purpose flour
- 1/2 cup whole-wheat flour
- 1 cup whole milk
- 1/2 cup water
- 1 tsp. active dry yeast
- 1 tsp. baking powder
- 1/2 tsp. salt
- 2 TB. sugar
- 2 cups Ashta Custard (recipe later in this chapter)
- 1/2 cup ground pistachios
- 1 cup Simple Syrup (recipe later in this chapter)

Directions:

1. In a large bowl, whisk together all-purpose flour, whole-wheat flour, whole milk, water, yeast, baking powder, salt, and sugar. Set aside for 30 minutes.

2. Preheat a nonstick griddle over low heat.

3. Spoon 3 tablespoons batter onto the griddle, and cook pancake for about 30 seconds or until bubbles form

along entire top of pancake. Do not flip over pancake. You're only browning the bottom.

4. Transfer pancake to a plate, and let cool while cooking remaining pancakes. Do not overlap the pancakes while letting them cool.

5. Form pancake into a pocket by folding pancake into a half-moon, and pinch together the edges, but only halfway up.

6. Spoon Ashta Custard into a piping bag or a zipper-lock plastic bag, snip off the corner, and squeeze about 2 tablespoons custard into each pancake pocket. Sprinkle custard with pistachios.

7. Serve pancakes chilled with Simple Syrup drizzled on top.

Pomegranate Granita With Lychee

Servings: 7

Cooking Time: 5 Minutes

Ingredients:

- 500 millimeters pomegranate juice, organic and sugar-free
- 1 cup water
- ½ cup lychee syrup
- 2 tablespoons lemon juice
- 4 mint leaves
- 1 cup fresh lychees, pitted and sliced

Directions:

1. Place all Ingredients: in a large pitcher.
2. Place inside the fridge to cool before serving.

Nutrition Info: Calories per serving: 96; Carbs: 23.8g; Protein: 0.4g; Fat: 0.4g

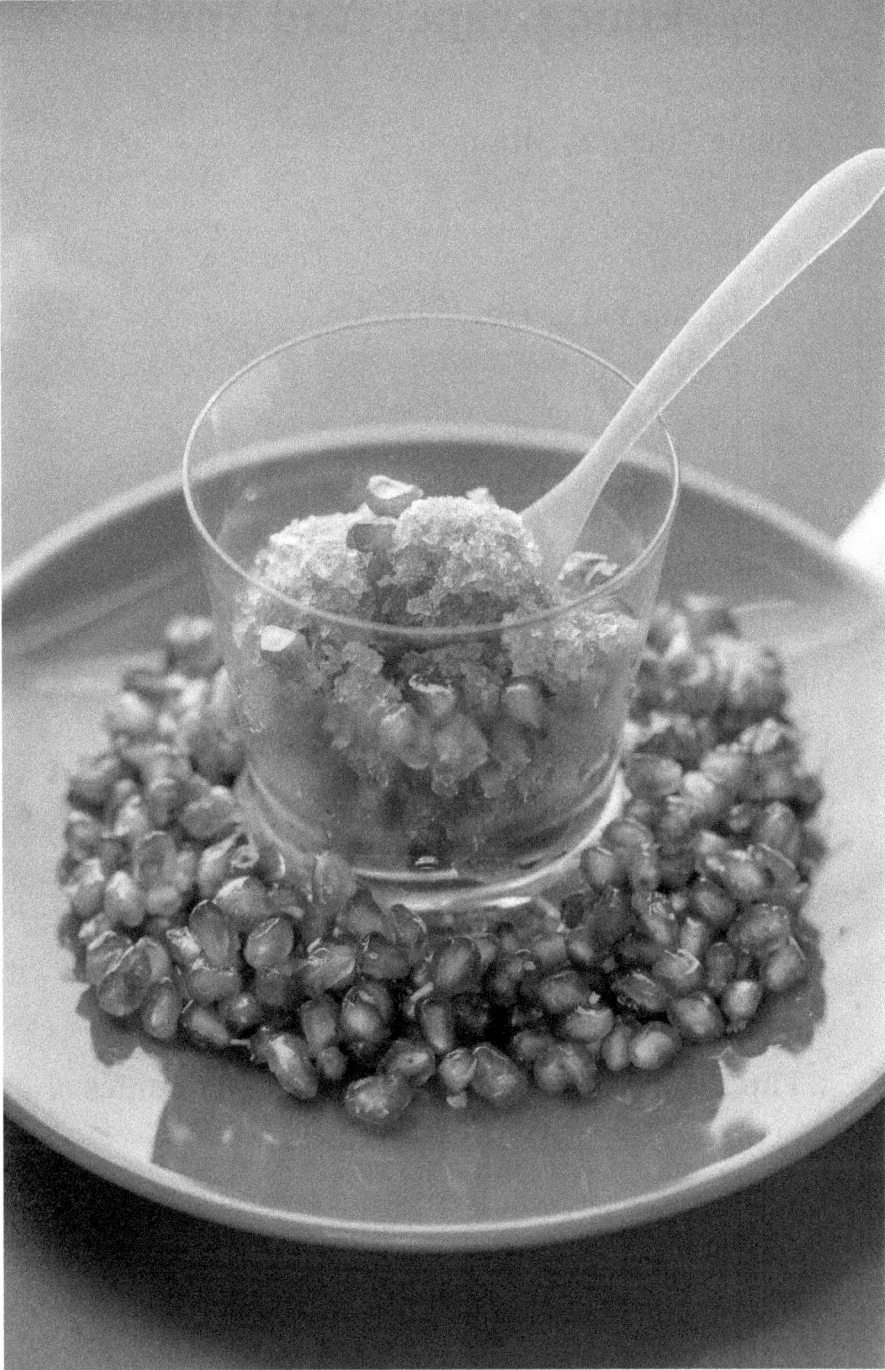

Lime Grapes And Apples

Servings: 2

Cooking Time: 25 Minutes

Ingredients:

- ½ cup red grapes
- 2 apples
- 1 teaspoon lime juice
- 1 teaspoon Erythritol
- 3 tablespoons water

Directions:

1. Line the baking tray with baking paper.

2. Then cut the apples on the halves and remove the seeds with the help of the scooper.

3. Cut the apple halves on 2 parts more.

4. Arrange all fruits in the tray in one layer, drizzle with water, and bake for 20 minutes at 375F.

5. Flip the fruits on another side after 10 minutes of cooking.

6. Then remove them from the oven and sprinkle with lime juice and Erythritol.

7. Return the fruits back in the oven and bake for 5 minutes more.

8. Serve the cooked dessert hot or warm.

Nutrition Info:Per Serving:calories 142, fat 0.4, fiber 5.7, carbs 40.1, protein 0.9

Mediterranean Baked Apples

Servings: 4

Cooking Time: 25 Minutes

Ingredients:

- 1.5 pounds apples, peeled and sliced
- Juice from ½ lemon
- A dash of cinnamon

Directions:

1. Preheat the oven to 250F.

2. Line a baking sheet with parchment paper then set aside.

3. In a medium bowl, apples with lemon juice and cinnamon.

4. Place the apples on the parchment paper-lined baking sheet.

5. Bake for 25 minutes until crisp.

Nutrition Info: Calories per serving: 90; Carbs: 23.9g; Protein: 0.5g; Fat: 0.3g

Poached Cherries

Servings: 5

Cooking Time: 10 Minutes

Ingredients:

- 1 pound fresh and sweet cherries, rinsed, pitted
- 3 strips (1x3 inches each) orange zest,
- 3 strips (1x3 inches each) lemon zest,
- 2/3 cup sugar
- 15 peppercorns
- 1/4 vanilla bean, split but not scraped
- 1 3/4 cups water

Directions:

1. In a saucepan, mix the water, citrus zest, sugar, peppercorns, and vanilla bean; bring to a boil, stirring until the sugar is dissolved. Add the cherries; simmer for about 10 minutes until the cherries are soft, but not falling apart. Skim any foam from the surface and let the poached cherries cool. Refrigerate with the poaching liquid. Before serving, strain the cherries.

Nutrition Info:Per Serving:170 cal., 1 g total fat (0 g sat. fat, 0 g mono fat, 0.5 g poly fat), 0 mg chol., 0 mg sodium, 42 g total carbs., and 2 g fiber.

Watermelon Salad

Servings: 6

Cooking Time: 0 Minutes

Ingredients:

- 14 oz watermelon
- 1 oz dark chocolate
- 3 tablespoons coconut cream
- 1 teaspoon Erythritol
- 2 kiwi, chopped
- 1 oz Feta cheese, crumbled

Directions:

1. Peel the watermelon and remove the seeds from it.
2. Chop the fruit and place in the salad bowl.
3. Add chopped kiwi and crumbled Feta. Stir the salad well.
 4. Then mix up together coconut cream and Erythritol.
5. Pour the cream mixture over the salad.
6. Then shave the chocolate over the salad with the help of the potato peeler.
7. The salad should be served immediately.

Nutrition Info:Per Serving:calories 90, fat 4.4, fiber 1.4, carbs 12.9, protein 1.9

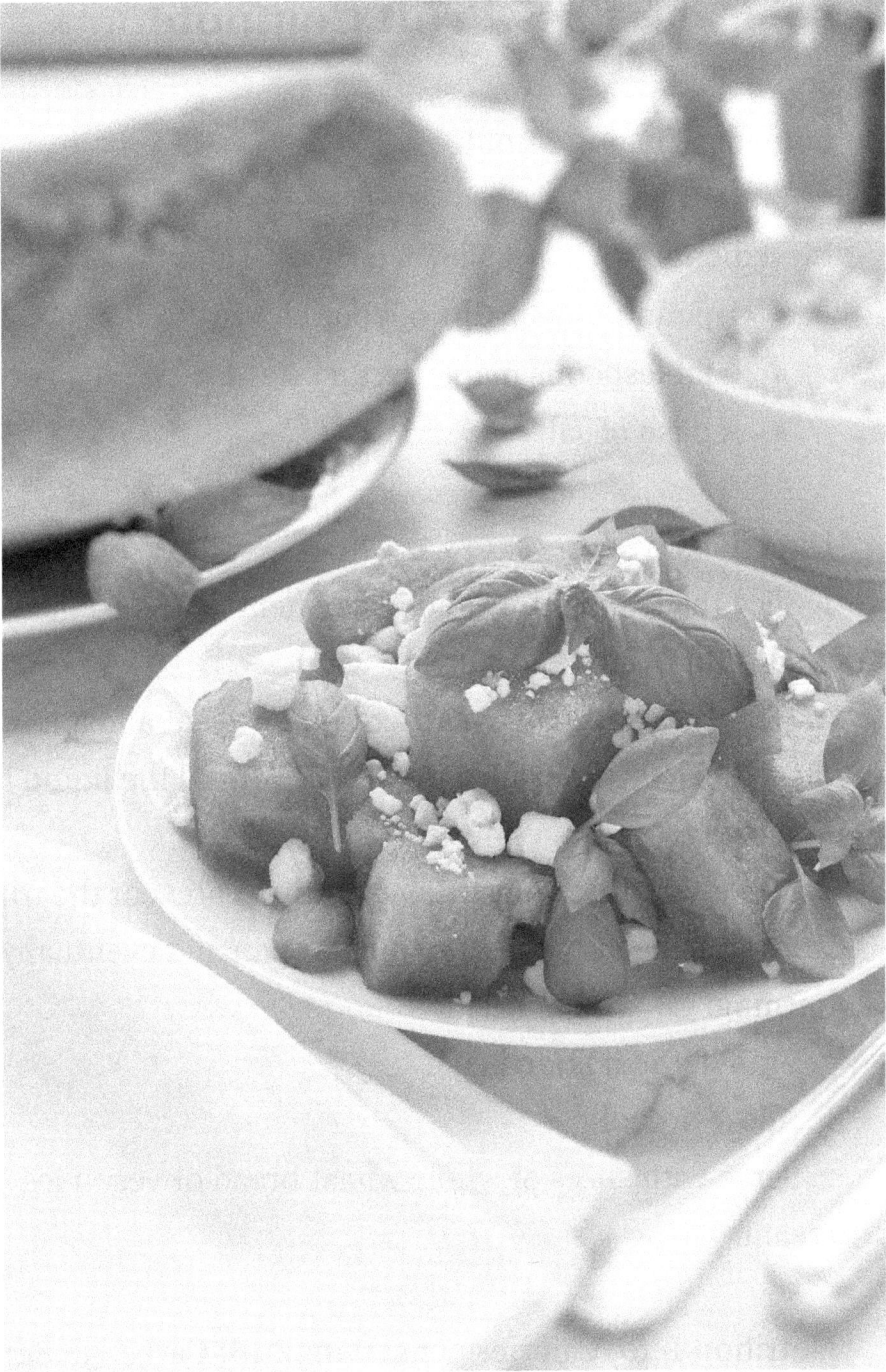

Easy Fruit Compote

Servings: 2

Cooking Time: 15 Minutes

Ingredients:

- 1-pound fresh fruits of your choice
- 2 tablespoons maple syrup
- A dash of salt

Directions:

1. Slice the fruits thinly and place them in a saucepan.

2. Add the honey and salt.

3. Heat the saucepan over medium low heat and allow the fruits to simmer for 15 minutes or until the liquid has reduced.

4. Make sure that you stir constantly to prevent the fruits from sticking at the bottom of your pan and eventually burning.

5. Transfer in a lidded jar.

6. Allow to cool.

7. Serve with slices of whole wheat bread or vegan ice cream.

Nutrition Info: Calories per serving:218; Carbs: 56.8g; Protein: 0.9g; Fat: 0.2g

Papaya Cream

Servings: 2

Cooking Time: 0 Minutes

Ingredients:

- 1 cup papaya, peeled and chopped
- 1 cup heavy cream
- 1 tablespoon stevia
- ½ teaspoon vanilla extract

Directions:

1. In a blender, combine the cream with the papaya and the other ingredients, pulse well, divide into cups and serve cold.

Nutrition Info: calories 182, fat 3.1, fiber 2.3, carbs 3.5, protein 2

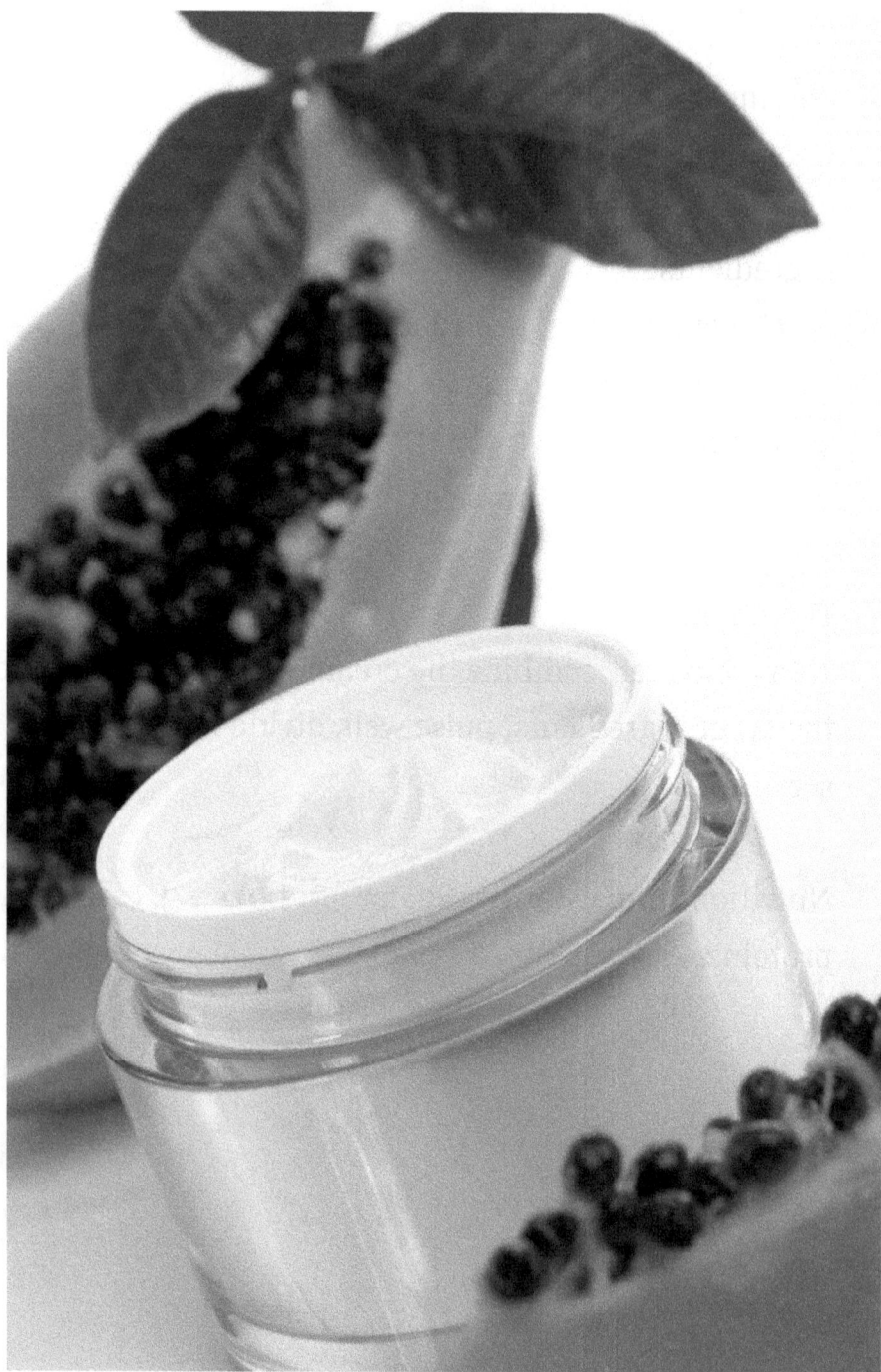

Minty Tart

Servings: 6

Cooking Time: 30 Minutes

Ingredients:

- 1 cup tart cherries, pitted
- 1 cup wheat flour, whole grain
- 1/3 cup butter, softened
- ½ teaspoon baking powder
- 1 tablespoon Erythritol
- ¼ teaspoon dried mint
- ¾ teaspoon salt

Directions:

1. Mix up together wheat flour and cutter.

2. Add baking powder and salt. Knead the soft dough.

3. Then place the dough in the freezer for 10 minutes.

4. When the dough is solid, remove it from the freezer and grate with the help of the grater. Place ¼ part of the grated dough in the freezer.

5. Sprinkle the springform pan with remaining dough and place tart
cherries on it.

6. Sprinkle the berries with Erythritol and dried mint and cover with ¼ part of dough from the freezer.

7. Bake the cake for 30 minutes at 365F. The cooked tart will have a golden brown surface.

Nutrition Info:Per Serving:calories 177, fat 10.4, fiber 0.9, carbs 21, protein 2.4

Orange-sesame Almond Tuiles

Servings: 20

Cooking Time: 45 Minutes

Ingredients:

- 3/4 cup unblanched or blanched sliced almonds
- 3 tablespoons orange juice, freshly squeezed
- 3 tablespoons (about 1 1/2 ounce) unsalted or salted butter
- 2 tablespoons white sesame seeds
- 10 tablespoons granulated sugar
- 1/8 cup whole-wheat flour
- 1/8 cup all-purpose flour
- 1 tablespoon toasted sesame oil
- 1 1/2 teaspoons black sesame seeds
- Grated zest of 1 orange, preferably organic

Directions:

1. In a small-sized saucepan, warm the butter, sesame oil, orange zest, orange juice, and sugar over low heat until the mixture is smooth. Remove from the heat, Stir the flour, almonds and the sesame seeds; let the batter rest for 1 hour at normal room temperature.

2. Preheat the oven to 375F. Line 2 pieces baking sheet with parchment paper.

3. Set a rolling pin on a folded dishtowel. Ready a wire rack.

4. Measuring by level tablespoons, drop batter into the prepared baking sheets, placing only 4 on each sheet and spacing them apart evenly.

5. With dampened fingers, slightly flatten the batter. Place one baking sheet in the oven, bake the tuiles for about 8 to 9 minutes, rotating the baking sheet halfway through baking, until the cookies are evenly browned. Let the cookies cool slightly for1 minute.

6. With a metal spatula, lift each cookie of the baking sheet and then drape
them over the rolling pin. Let them cool in the rolling pin and then transfer to a wire rack. Repeat the process with the remaining batter. Serve the tuiles a few hours after baking.

Nutrition Info:Per Serving:78 cal., 4.7 g total fat (1.4 g sat. fat), 5 mg chol., 13 mg sodium, 39 mg pto., 8.6 g total carbs., 0.7 g fiber, 6.4 g sugar, and 1.1 g protein.

Strawberry Ice Cream

Servings: 6

Cooking Time: 1 ¼ Hours

Ingredients:

- 1 pound strawberries, hulled
- 1 cup Greek yogurt
- 1 cup heavy cream
- 3 tablespoons honey
- 1 teaspoon lime zest

Directions:

1. Combine all the ingredients in a blender and pulse until well mixed and smooth.

2. Pour the mixture into your ice cream machine and churn for 1 hour or according to your machine's instructions.

3. Serve the ice cream right away.

Nutrition Info: Per Serving:Calories:150 Fat:8.3g Protein:4.3g Carbohydrates:16.4g

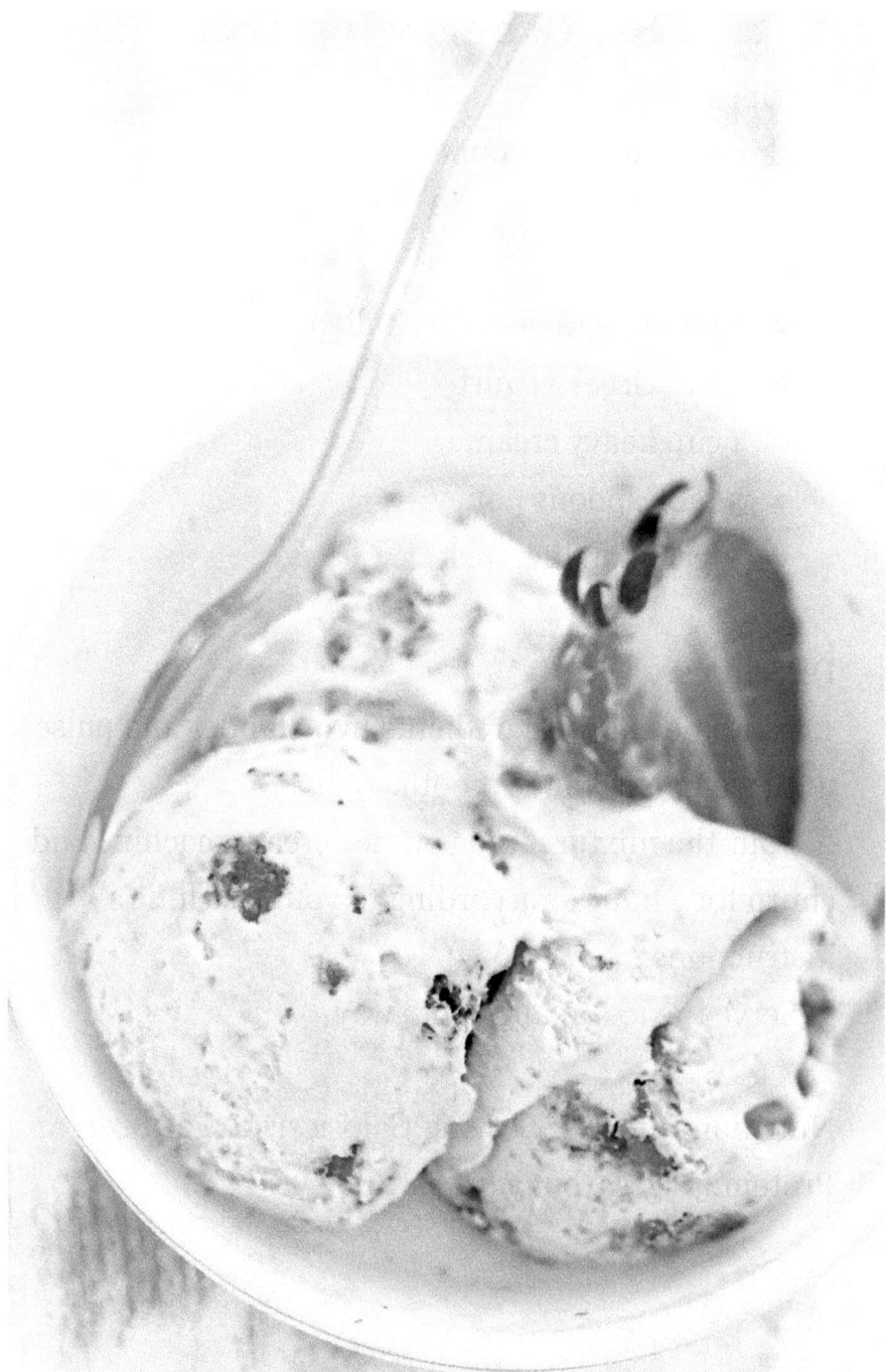

Creamy Strawberries

Servings: 4

Cooking Time: 5 Minutes

Ingredients:

- 6 tablespoons almond butter
- 1 tablespoon Erythritol
- 1 cup milk
- 1 teaspoon vanilla extract
- 1 cup strawberries, sliced

Directions:

1. Pour milk in the saucepan.

2. Add Erythritol, vanilla extract, and almond butter.

3. With the help of the hand mixer mix up the liquid until smooth and bring it to boil.

4. Then remove the mixture from the heat and let it cool.

5. The cooled mixture will be thick.

6. Put the strawberries in the serving glasses and top with the thick almond butter dip.

Nutrition Info:Per Serving:calories 192, fat 14.9, fiber 3.1, carbs 10.4, protein 7.3

Greek Yogurt Pie

Servings: 8

Cooking Time: 1 Hour

Ingredients:

- 1 package phyllo dough sheets
- 4 cups plain yogurt
- 4 eggs
- ½ cup white sugar
- 1 teaspoon vanilla extract
- 1 teaspoon lemon zest
- 1 teaspoon orange zest

Directions:

1. Mix the yogurt, eggs, sugar, vanilla and citrus zest in a bowl.
2. Layer 2 phyllo sheets in a deep dish baking pan then pour a few tablespoons of yogurt mixture over the dough.
3. Continue layering the phyllo dough and yogurt in the pan.
4. Bake in the preheated oven at 350F for 40 minutes.
5. Allow the pie to cool down before serving.

Nutrition Info: Per Serving:Calories:175 Fat:3.8g Protein:9.9g Carbohydrates:22.7g

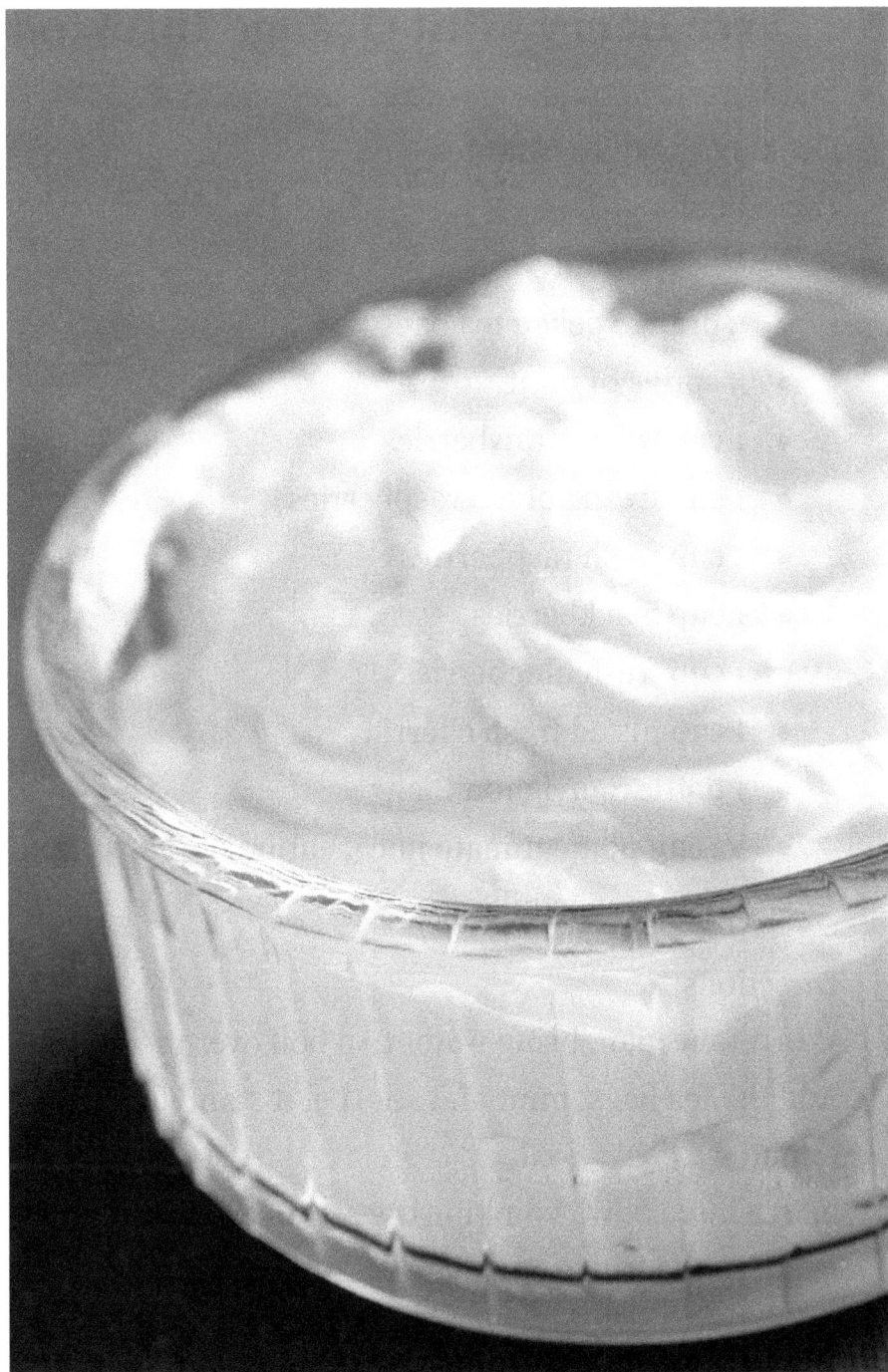

Five Berry Mint Orange Infusion

Servings: 12

Cooking Time: 10 Minutes

Ingredients:

- ½ cup water
- 3 orange pekoe tea bags
- 3 sprigs of mint
- 1 cup fresh strawberries
- 1 cup fresh golden raspberries
- 1 cup fresh raspberries
- 1 cup blackberries
- 1 cup fresh blueberries
- 1 cup pitted fresh cherries
- 1 bottle Sauvignon Blanc
- ½ cup pomegranate juice, natural
- 1 teaspoon vanilla

Directions:

1. In a saucepan, bring water to a boil over medium heat. Add the tea bags, mint and stir. Let it stand for 10 minutes.
2. In a large bowl, combine the rest of the ingredients.
3. Put in the fridge to chill for at least 3 hours.

Nutrition Info: Calories per serving: 140; Carbs: 32.1g; Protein: 1.2g; Fat: 1.5g

Cocoa Yogurt Mix

Servings: 2

Cooking Time: 0 Minutes

Ingredients:

- 1 tablespoon cocoa powder
- ¼ cup strawberries, chopped
- ¾ cup Greek yogurt
- 5 drops vanilla stevia

Directions:

1. In a bowl, mix the yogurt with the cocoa, strawberries and the stevia and whisk well.
2. Divide the mix into bowls and serve.

Nutrition Info: calories 200, fat 8, fiber 3.4, carbs 7.6, protein 4.3

Almond Rice Dessert

Servings: 4

Cooking Time: 20 Minutes

Ingredients:

- 1 cup white rice
- 2 cups almond milk
- 1 cup almonds, chopped
- ½ cup stevia
- 1 tablespoon cinnamon powder
- ½ cup pomegranate seeds

Directions:

1. In a pot, mix the rice with the milk and stevia, bring to a simmer and cook for 20 minutes, stirring often.
2. Add the rest of the ingredients, stir, divide into bowls and serve.

Nutrition Info: calories 234, fat 9.5, fiber 3.4, carbs 12.4, protein 6.

Frozen Strawberry Greek Yogurt

Servings: 16

Cooking Time: 15 Minutes

Ingredients:

- 3 cups Greek yogurt, plain, low-fat (2%)
- 2 teaspoons vanilla
- 1/8 teaspoon salt
- 1/4 cup freshly squeezed lemon juice
- 1 cup sugar
- 1 cup strawberries, sliced

Directions:

1. In a medium-sized bowl, except for the strawberries, combine the rest of the ingredients; whisking until the mixture is smooth.

2. Transfer the yogurt into a 1 1/2 or 2-quart ice cream make and freeze according to the manufacturer's direction, adding the strawberry slices for the last minute. Transfer into an airtight container and freeze for about 2-4 hours. Before serving, let stand for 15 minutes at room temperature.

Nutrition Info:Per Serving:86 cal., 1 g total fat (1 g sat. fat), 3 mg chol., 16g carbs., 0 g fiber, 15 g sugar, and 4 g protein.

Almond Peaches Mix

Servings: 4

Cooking Time: 10 Minutes

Ingredients:

- 1/3 cup almonds, toasted
- 1/3 cup pistachios, toasted
- 1 teaspoon mint, chopped
- ½ cup coconut water
- 1 teaspoon lemon zest, grated
- 4 peaches, halved
- 2 tablespoons stevia

Directions:

1. In a pan, combine the peaches with the stevia and the rest of the ingredients, simmer over medium heat for 10 minutes, divide into bowls and serve cold.

Nutrition Info: calories 135, fat 4.1, fiber 3.8, carbs 4.1, protein 2.3

Raisin Pecan Baked Apples

Servings: 6

Cooking Time: 4 Minutes

Ingredients:

- 6 apples, cored and cut into wedges
- 1 cup red wine
- 1/4 cup pecans, chopped
- 1/4 cup raisins
- 1/4 tsp nutmeg
- 1 tsp cinnamon
- 1/3 cup honey

Directions:

1. Add all ingredients into the instant pot and stir well.

2. Seal pot with lid and cook on high for 4 minutes.

3. Once done, allow to release pressure naturally for 10 minutes then release remaining using quick release. Remove lid.

4. Stir well and serve.

Nutrition Info: Calories 229 Fat 0.9 g Carbohydrates 52.6 g Sugar 42.6 g Protein 1 g Cholesterol 0 mg

Walnuts Cake

Servings: 4

Cooking Time: 40 Minutes

Ingredients:

- ½ pound walnuts, minced
- Zest of 1 orange, grated
- 1 and ¼ cups stevia
- eggs, whisked
- 1 teaspoon almond extract
- 1 and ½ cup almond flour
- 1 teaspoon baking soda

Directions:

1. In a bowl, combine the walnuts with the orange zest and the other ingredients, whisk well and pour into a cake pan lined with parchment paper.
2. Introduce in the oven at 350 degrees F, bake for 40 minutes, cool down, slice and serve

.

Nutrition Info: calories 205, fat 14.1, fiber 7.8, carbs 9.1, protein 3.4

Notes

www.ingramcontent.com/pod-product-compliance
Lightning Source LLC
Chambersburg PA
CBHW050759030426
42336CB00012B/1878